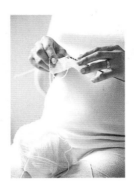

my pregnancy journal

_____

_____

_____

_____

_____

_____

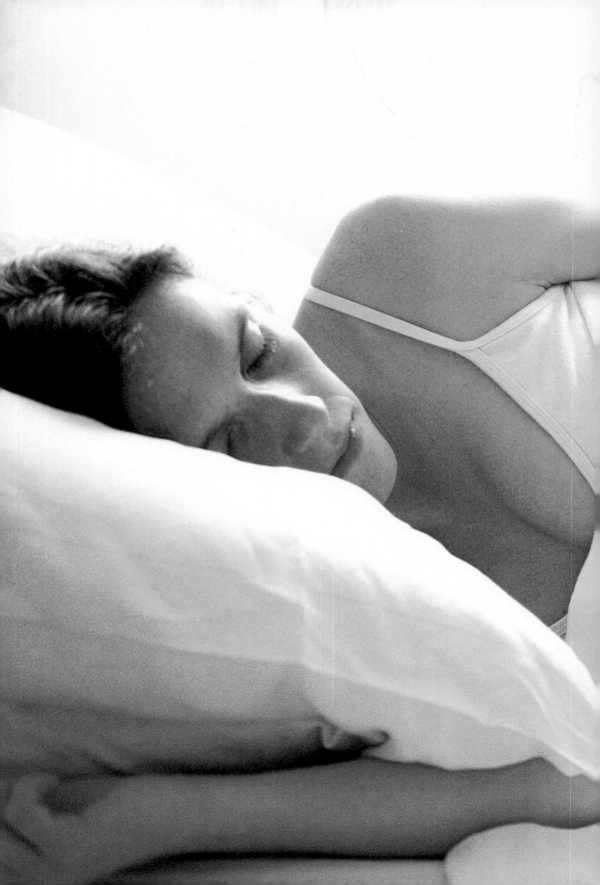

my pregnancy journal

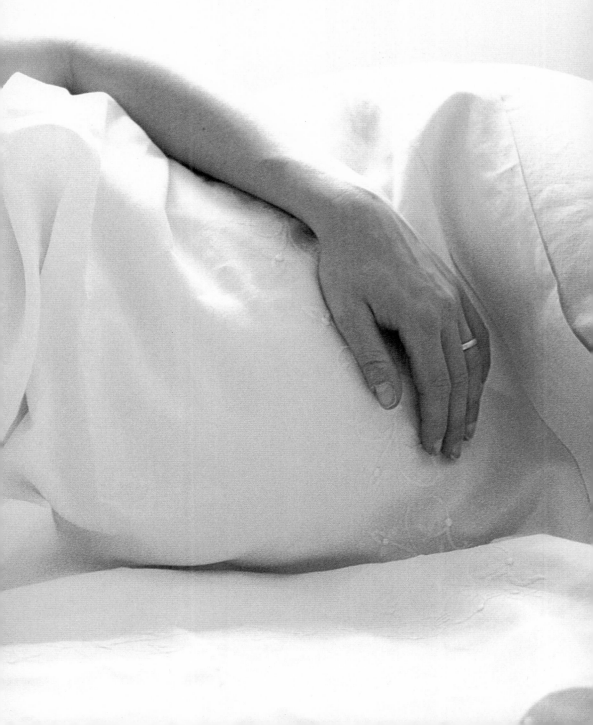

contents

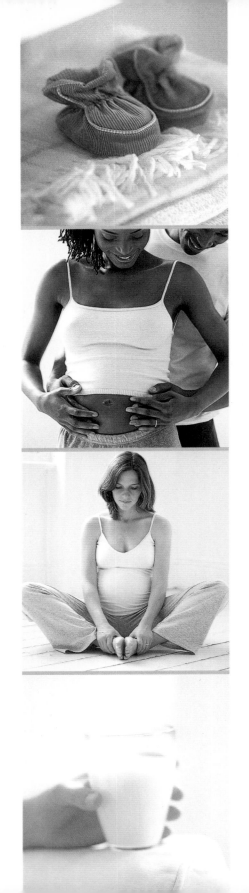

introduction

Bringing a child into the world is one of the most rewarding things you will ever do. It could also be one of the most life-changing experiences you will ever have. Throughout your pregnancy you will go through all sorts of physical and emotional changes as you and your body prepare for the arrival of your little bundle of joy—it is a magical time.

Use this journal to record every precious moment of your pregnancy—from the first sight of your baby on an ultrasound scan and the thrill of the first kick to unusual food cravings and swollen ankles. Store cards and ultrasound scan photos in the pockets provided in each section to build up a complete and unique memento of your pregnancy and your baby's birth, which you and your partner can enjoy looking back at time and time again. It will also be a delightful keepsake for you to share with your child once she or he is older.

My pregnancy calendar

The average length of a pregnancy is 280 days (40 weeks) from the start of the last menstrual period. This week-by-week calendar is 42 weeks long to allow for the possibility of you going up to two weeks overdue. Use it to keep track of any important dates during your pregnancy.

weeks 1 and 2

_____

_____

_____

weeks 3 and 4

_____

_____

_____

week 5

_____

_____

_____

_____

_____

_____

week 6

_____

_____

_____

_____

_____

_____

week 7

_____

_____

_____

_____

_____

_____

week 8

_____

_____

_____

_____

_____

_____

week 9

_____

_____

_____

_____

_____

_____

week 10

_____

_____

_____

_____

_____

_____

week 11

_____

_____

_____

_____

_____

_____

week 12

_____

_____

_____

_____

_____

_____

week 13

_____
_____
_____
_____
_____
_____
_____

week 14

_____
_____
_____
_____
_____
_____
_____

week 15

_____
_____
_____
_____
_____
_____
_____

week 16

_____
_____
_____
_____
_____
_____
_____

week 17

_____
_____
_____
_____
_____
_____
_____

week 18

_____
_____
_____
_____
_____
_____
_____

week 19

_____
_____
_____
_____
_____
_____
_____

week 20

_____
_____
_____
_____
_____
_____
_____

week 21

_____
_____
_____
_____
_____
_____
_____

week 22

_____
_____
_____
_____
_____
_____
_____

week 23

week 24

week 25

week 26

week 27

week 28

week 29

week 30

week 31

week 32

week 33

_____
_____
_____
_____
_____
_____
_____

week 34

_____
_____
_____
_____
_____
_____
_____

week 35

_____
_____
_____
_____
_____
_____
_____

week 36

_____
_____
_____
_____
_____
_____
_____

week 37

_____
_____
_____
_____
_____
_____
_____

week 38

_____
_____
_____
_____
_____
_____
_____

week 39

_____
_____
_____
_____
_____
_____

week 40

_____
_____
_____
_____
_____
_____

week 41

_____
_____
_____
_____
_____
_____

week 42

_____
_____
_____
_____
_____
_____

My emergency telephone numbers

Name	Number

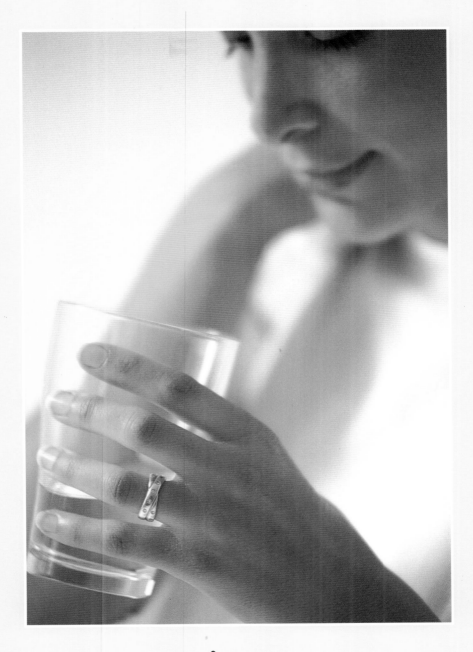

preparing for pregnancy

THINKING IT THROUGH

Deciding to bring a new baby into the world is probably the most important decision you and your partner will ever make. But in the excitement of imagining what it will be like to have this amazing new person created by the two of you, it is easy to lose sight of the enormous responsibility involved in making sure he has the best possible start in life.

You and your partner need to consider carefully the impact that this life-changing decision will have on your relationship together, as well as on both of your lives in general. Each baby is unique and will have his own special set of demands. You need to make sure that both of you can meet these demands, whatever they are. That way you can ensure that this truly is the beginning of the most rewarding relationship for all of you.

"A mother's love endures through all."

Washington Irving (1783—1859)

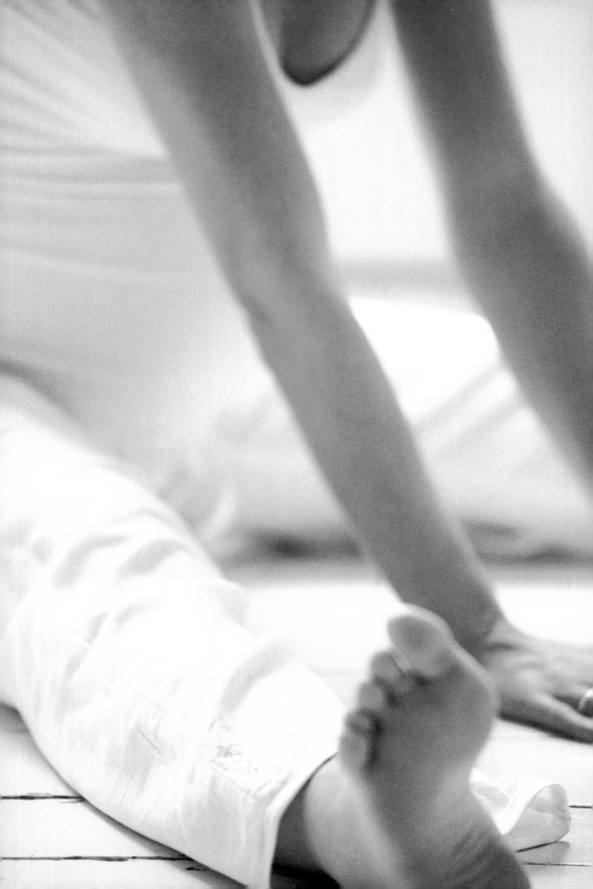

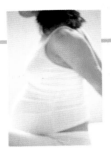

Fitness

Before you get pregnant—and throughout your pregnancy—you should try to make sure that you are reasonably fit. It is also a good idea not to be either overweight or underweight, as both conditions can impede your chances of conception and cause discomfort during pregnancy. Pregnancy places extra demands on your body and although it's built to adapt so that you can carry on as much as normal, women who are reasonably fit and of normal weight usually have an easier pregnancy. And an easier pregnancy means you can enjoy this time much more and give your baby the best possible start in life.

If you're not already doing regular exercise prior to your pregnancy, check with your doctor or midwife before starting a new regimen. Your local gym and swimming pool may run classes especially tailored for pregnant women. Otherwise, walking is particularly good exercise when pregnant.

It is important to do pelvic floor exercises (also known as Kegel exercises) throughout your pregnancy. If you are not sure how to do these then ask your doctor or midwife for instructions. Exercising these muscles will help to support the weight of your baby as she grows. Strong pelvic floor muscles will also help to reduce your chances of suffering from stress incontinence during pregnancy and after birth.

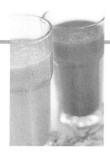

Healthy eating

Although you should always have a healthy diet and eat at least five daily servings of fruit and vegetables, this is particularly important now that you are pregnant. You should also make sure you are eating a balanced diet with sufficient carbohydrates, protein, fat, minerals, and vitamins—as well as plenty of fiber to help prevent constipation (a common complaint during pregnancy).

It is recommended that all women of childbearing age take 400mcg of folic acid (vitamin B9) daily and that this is increased to 600mcg daily when pregnant. Folic acid can be consumed through the diet—dark green, leafy vegetables are good sources, and in the United States bread, pasta and grains are fortified with the vitamin—but most women take a supplement. In some cases you may be given a prescription for it and other vitamins and minerals by your doctor once he is aware you are pregnant.

Foods to avoid in pregnancy

There are certain foods that you should cut out as soon as you suspect you may be pregnant because they may cause harm to your unborn baby. Among others, these include cooked foods that are subsequently chilled and then eaten cold—such as paté—unless they are pasteurized; unpasteurized dairy produce such as soft and blue-veined cheese; undercooked meat; foods with raw or undercooked eggs; raw shellfish or fish; and giblets or other organ meat. Certain fatty fish have been found to contain high levels of mercury or other contaminants. It is also advisable to cut down on your caffeine intake, stop alcohol consumption, and stop smoking. The Food and Drug Administration has helpful information about nutrition and food safety on their website (www.fda.gov) as does the Department of Agriculture (www.usda.gov). You might like to make a list below of the foods that you need to avoid.

_____

_____

_____

_____

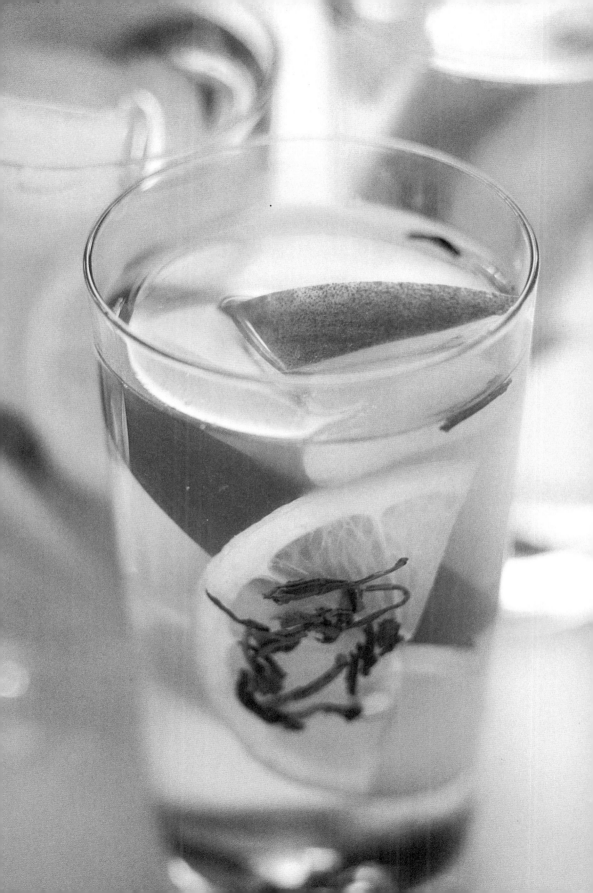

My medical history

Date of birth

10-2-1989

First day of last menstrual period

(known as LMP) 10-3-2015

Date pregnancy confirmed

Any childhood illnesses

None

Time spent in hospital/operations

None

Blood type

Allergies

None

Immunizations

Any hereditary illnesses

NO

Family history of twins

yes

Height 5'7"

Weight (before pregnancy)

108

Blood pressure

116/68

Other details

My partner's medical history

Any childhood illnesses

NONE

Time spent in hospital/operations

Blood type

Allergies

Immunizations

Any hereditary illnesses

Family history of twins

Other details

"Wealth and children are the adornment of life."

The Koran

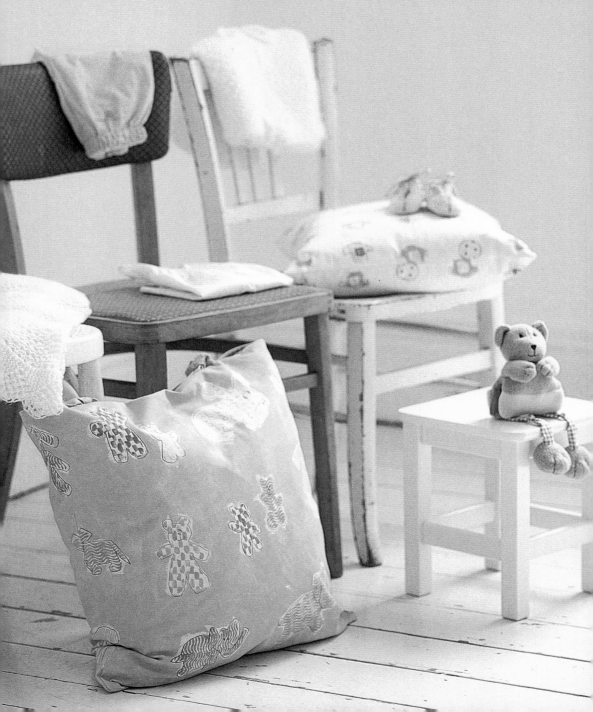

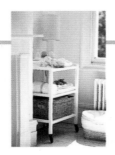

Budgeting for baby

A baby can cost a lot more money than you may at first think, but with some realistic budgeting it needn't put too much of a strain on your finances. Still, certain issues need to be addressed, such as what maternity benefits you are entitled to; whether you or your partner stop working; and what items you feel are essential to buy for the nursery. List below your monthly expenditure and income. Look at ways your spending could be reduced, and then plan for the future with a realistic budget.

Monthly expenditure	**Monthly earnings**
Mortgage/rent $1,000	My wages
Gas	My partner's wages
Electricity	Other
Water	
Telephone $70	
Credit cards	
Loan repayments —	
Travel costs $20/WK	
Car	
Insurance $115	
Foods $100	
Other	

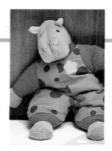

Childcare

Before having a baby talk to your partner about how you both feel about childcare. After all, while you may intend to continue with your career as soon as possible, he may feel that his child should be cared for by you for the first few years of her life. And if one of you does want to be your baby's primary caregiver, consider what impact stopping work or cutting back on hours would have on your monthly earnings.

Do I want to return to work after my baby's born?

yes

Does my partner want to keep working?

yes

How do I feel about childcare?

I prefer home Setting daycares

How does my partner feel about childcare?

What nurseries or babysitters are available in our area and how much do these cost?

Is there a waiting list?

Is there a member of family who could help with the day care?

yes

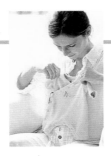

Preparing the nursery

One of the most fun aspects of preparing for your new arrival is getting the nursery ready. There are so many lovely items to choose from and you and your partner will get great pleasure out of creating the perfect environment for your baby.

The following list should help you work out what items you both feel are essential, and what other things you'd buy if money were no object. Fill in the prices of all the things you need to buy, then after you've bought these essentials you can see how many other pieces your budget will stretch to!

If you have friends or relatives who already have children, see if you can borrow some of the more expensive items, like a crib, from them. To keep an accurate record of items you have borrowed turn to page 63.

Item	Price
Crib	
Mattress	
Cradle or basket	
Bedding	
Changing pad	
Changing table	
Drawers	
Rocking or armchair (for feeding)	
Shelves	
Wardrobe	
Toy box	
Baby monitors	
Other	

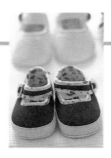

Notes

_____

_____

_____

_____

_____

_____

_____

_____

_____

_____

_____

_____

_____

_____

_____

_____

_____

_____

_____

_____

_____

_____

_____

_____

_____

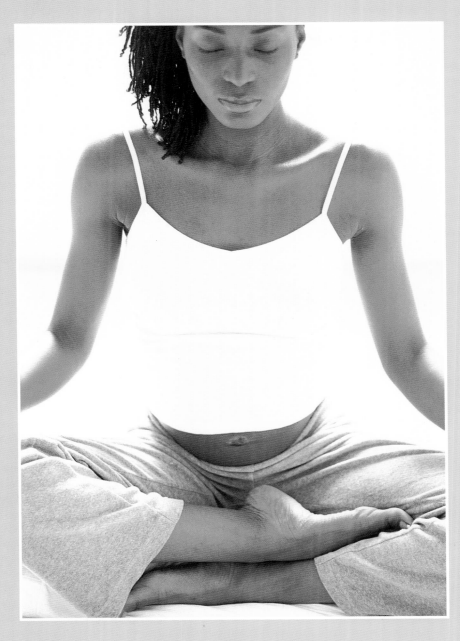

care and classes

Contacts

Make a note of the contact details of the medical personnel and other people you may need to get hold of during your pregnancy so you know where to find them when you need them. It might be useful for your partner to have a copy of these details, too.

My obstetrician's name is: _____

Address: _____

_____

_____

Telephone number: _____

My midwife's name is: _____

_____

Telephone number: _____

_____

My birthing class instructor's name is: _____

_____

Telephone number: _____

_____

My hospital's address is: _____

_____

_____

_____

_____

Telephone number: _____

_____

The labor ward telephone number is: _____

_____

Local taxi telephone number is: _____

_____

My birth partner's telephone numbers are: _____

_____

_____

_____

My insurance company's telephone number is: _____

_____

Any other important numbers: _____

_____

_____

_____

_____

_____

_____

_____

_____

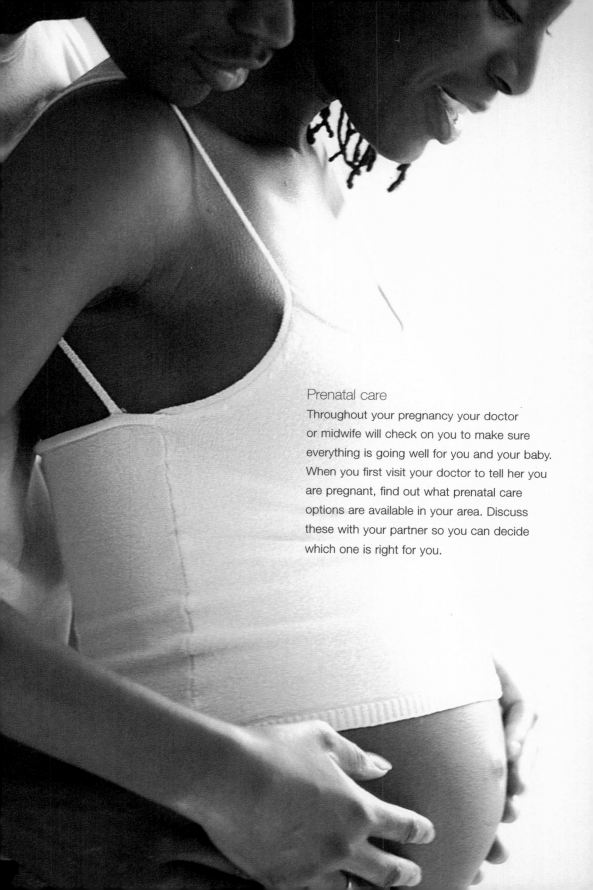

Prenatal care

Throughout your pregnancy your doctor
or midwife will check on you to make sure
everything is going well for you and your baby.
When you first visit your doctor to tell her you
are pregnant, find out what prenatal care
options are available in your area. Discuss
these with your partner so you can decide
which one is right for you.

Notes

_____
_____
_____
_____
_____
_____
_____
_____
_____
_____
_____
_____
_____
_____
_____
_____
_____
_____
_____
_____
_____
_____
_____
_____
_____
_____

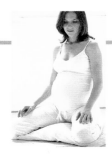

Prenatal visits

At each prenatal visit your doctor will check your blood pressure and test your urine for protein and glucose. As your pregnancy develops she will start to listen to your baby's heartbeat, and check his size and position. Towards the end of your pregnancy your visits will become more frequent.

Before each appointment think about any concerns you have and write down any questions you want to ask so you don't forget to ask her once you're at your appointment. Also, make a note of any symptoms you want to discuss with her. However, if you are feeling ill you should make an appointment to see your doctor.

Below is just a selection of things that may be bothering you. You can keep a comprehensive list of your own queries on pages 32—39 and fill in the answers after each appointment.

How do I contact you between visits if I have any concerns?

Can I bring my partner to my prenatal appointments?

Can I bring my partner to my ultrasound scan appointments?

Can I buy copies of the ultrasound scan photos?

What tests will I be offered during my pregnancy?

How accurate are these tests?

What risks do they carry to me and to my baby?

What prenatal class options are there in my local area?

What are my birthing options?

When can we have a tour of the labor ward?

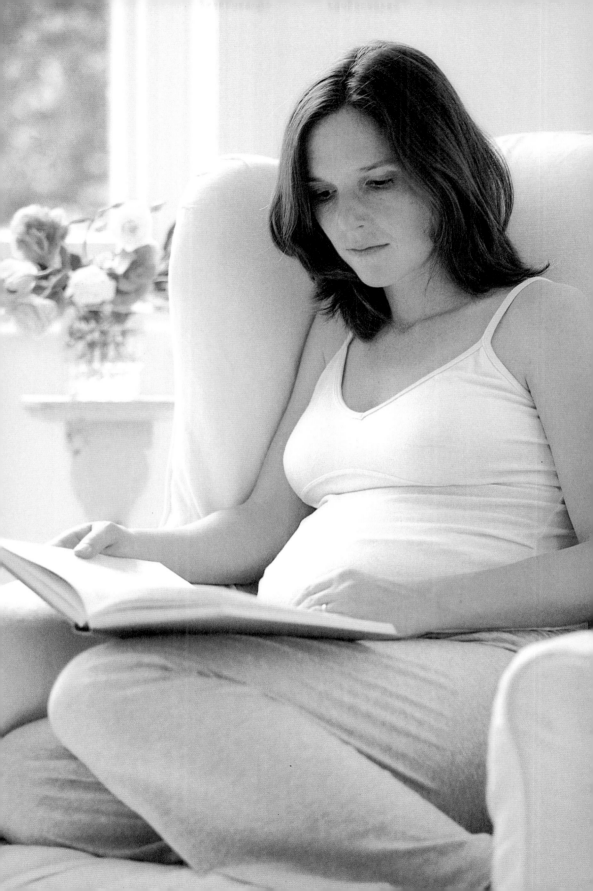

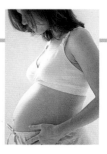

Notes on prenatal questions

_____

_____

_____

_____

_____

_____

_____

_____

_____

_____

_____

_____

_____

_____

_____

_____

_____

_____

_____

_____

_____

_____

_____

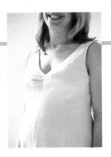

Notes on prenatal questions

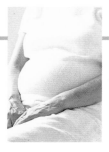

Notes on prenatal questions

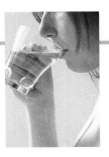

Notes on prenatal questions

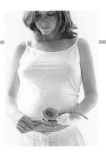

Notes on prenatal questions

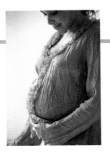

Notes on prenatal questions

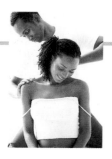

Notes on prenatal questions

_____

_____

_____

_____

_____

_____

_____

_____

_____

_____

_____

_____

_____

_____

_____

_____

_____

_____

_____

_____

_____

_____

_____

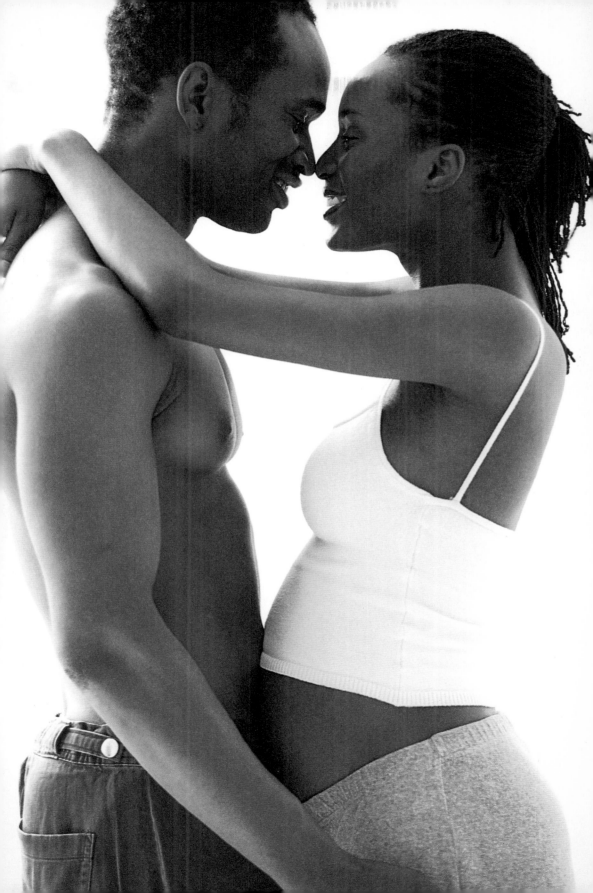

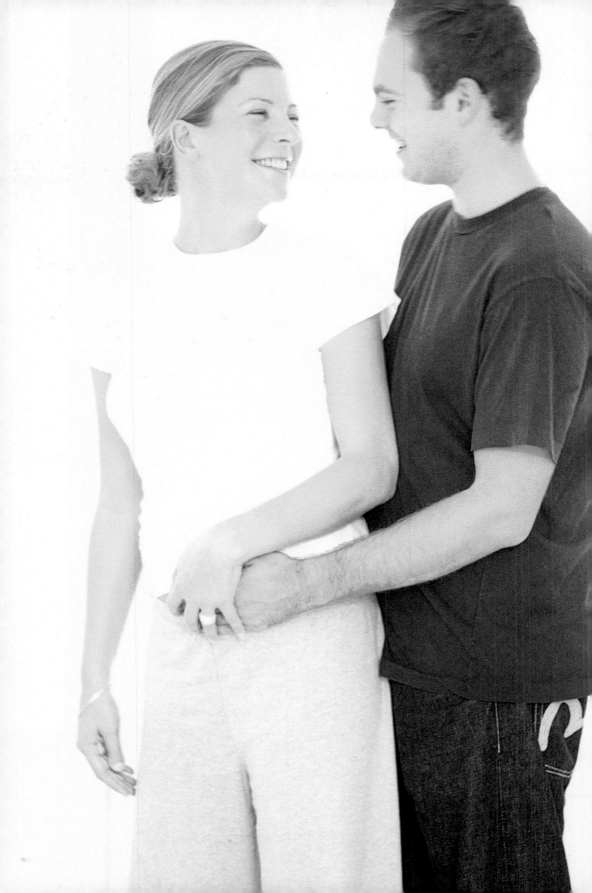

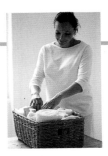

Birthing or parenting classes

Your hospital will probably offer you birthing or parenting classes, and it's a good idea to sign up for these. As well as providing you with invaluable information about pregnancy, labor, and looking after a newborn, they can be a great way to meet other moms-to-be in your area.

Your doctor or hospital should be able to give you a list of classes. Some classes are only for women; others will encourage you to bring your partner—make sure you attend the one that best suits your needs. Keep a note of all the things you've learned so you can refer to them and share them with your partner if he wasn't there with you.

Notes on birthing or parenting classes

_____

_____

_____

_____

_____

_____

_____

_____

_____

_____

_____

_____

_____

_____

_____

_____

_____

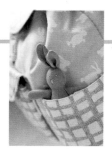

Notes on birthing or parenting classes

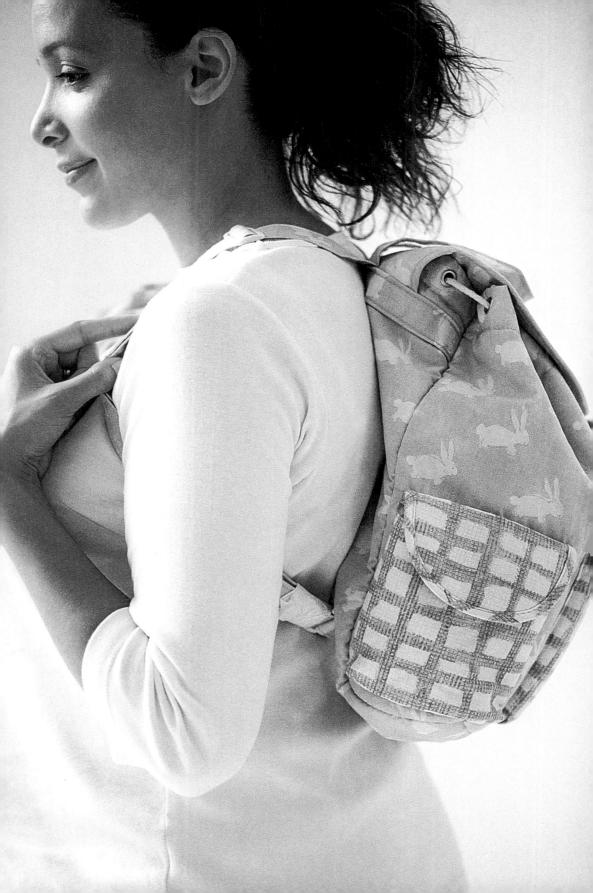

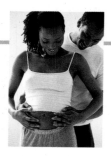

Notes on birthing or parenting classes
_____

_____

_____

_____

_____

_____

_____

_____

_____

_____

_____

_____

_____

_____

_____

_____

_____

_____

_____

_____

_____

_____

_____

_____

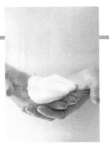

Notes on birthing or parenting classes

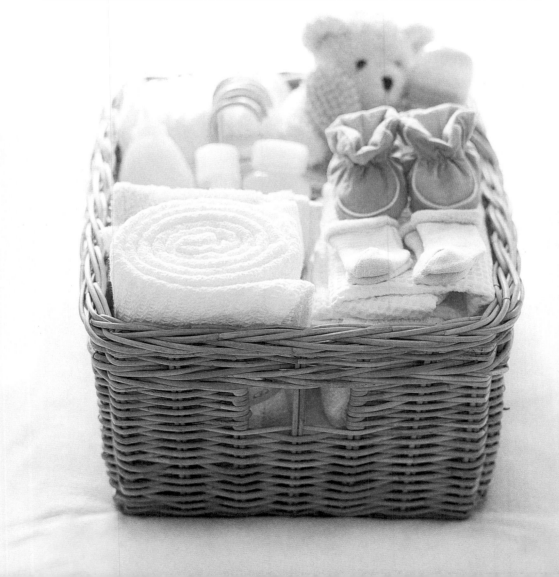

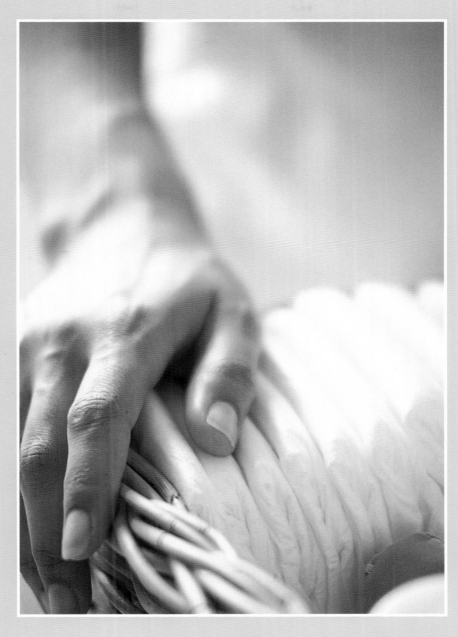

preparing for baby

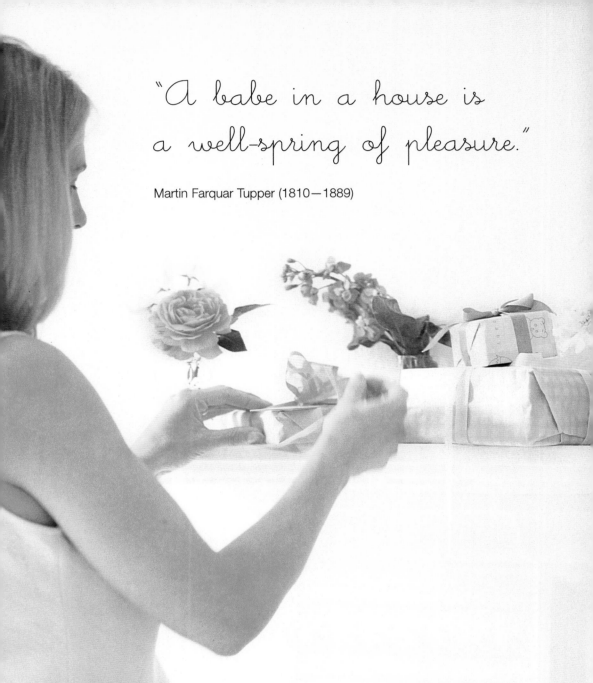

"A babe in a house is a well-spring of pleasure."

Martin Farquar Tupper (1810—1889)

PREPARING FOR THE NEW ARRIVAL

There is more than one reason why pregnancy lasts for nine months. It isn't just so your baby can develop properly, it's also so you have enough time to prepare for the new addition! Make the most of this time to get yourself ready both mentally and physically. Being prepared will remove some of the pressures you may feel about your baby's imminent arrival. So draw up a short-list of your favorite names, put together a checklist of what you need to buy for your baby, and get the nursery ready so when he finally arrives everything is ready for him.

Our favorite boys' names	Why we like them
Dylan	
Austin	

Short-list

Our final choice

Our favorite girls' names	Why we like them
~~Matthews~~	
Charlotte	
Alice	
Amelia	
Madeline	

Short-list

Our final choice

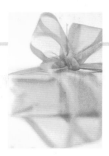

The baby shower

Given by
_____

_____

Where
_____

_____

_____

_____

_____

When
_____

_____

Who came?
_____

_____

_____

_____

_____

_____

_____

_____

_____

_____

_____

_____

_____

_____

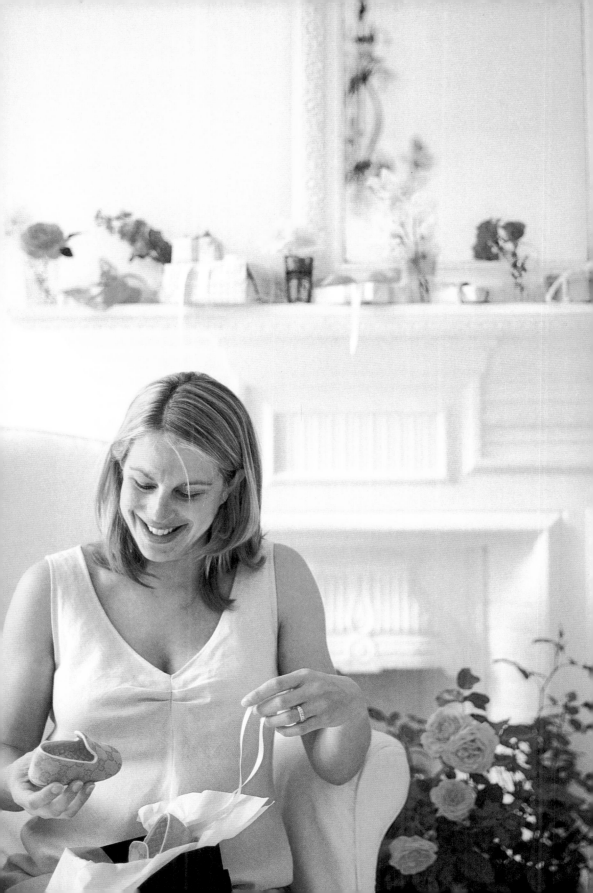

The gifts   From whom

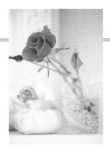

Special messages for the baby and the mom-to-be

Message   From whom

_____   _____

_____   _____

_____   _____

_____   _____

_____   _____

_____   _____

_____   _____

_____   _____

_____   _____

_____   _____

_____   _____

_____   _____

_____   _____

_____   _____

_____   _____

_____   _____

_____   _____

_____   _____

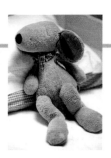

Decorating the nursery

The colors we like

_____

_____

_____

_____

The paint, paper, and fabric we chose

_____

_____

_____

_____

The furniture we chose

_____

_____

_____

_____

The finishing touches

_____

_____

_____

Stick fabric and wallpaper samples here

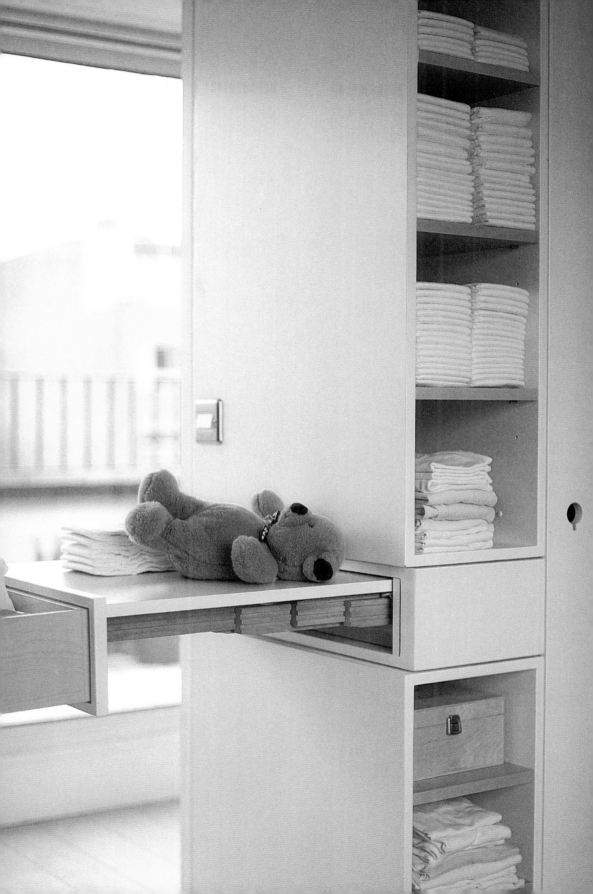

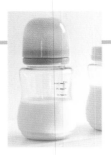

What I need to buy checklist

Crib

Mattress

Cradle or basket

Stand

Bedding

Changing pad

Changing table

Baby monitor

Bottles

Sterilizer

Baby bathtub

Baby carriage/stroller

Car seat

Baby carrier/sling

Baby clothes (see page 60 for more details)

Diapers

Blanket

Baby toiletries

Drawers

Wardrobe

Bookcase

Shelves

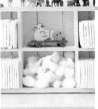

Other items

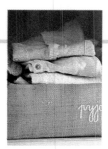

Baby clothes checklist

3—6 cotton footies

2—4 T-shirt cotton onesies

2—4 long-sleeve cotton onesies

2—4 short-sleeve cotton T-shirts

2—4 long-sleeve cotton T-shirts

1—2 two-piece outfits

1 cardigan

4—6 pairs of socks

2 pairs of slip-on bootees

2 washable bibs

1 hat

1 pair of shoes (optional)

For babies born in the winter:

1 pair of gloves or mittens

1 snowsuit

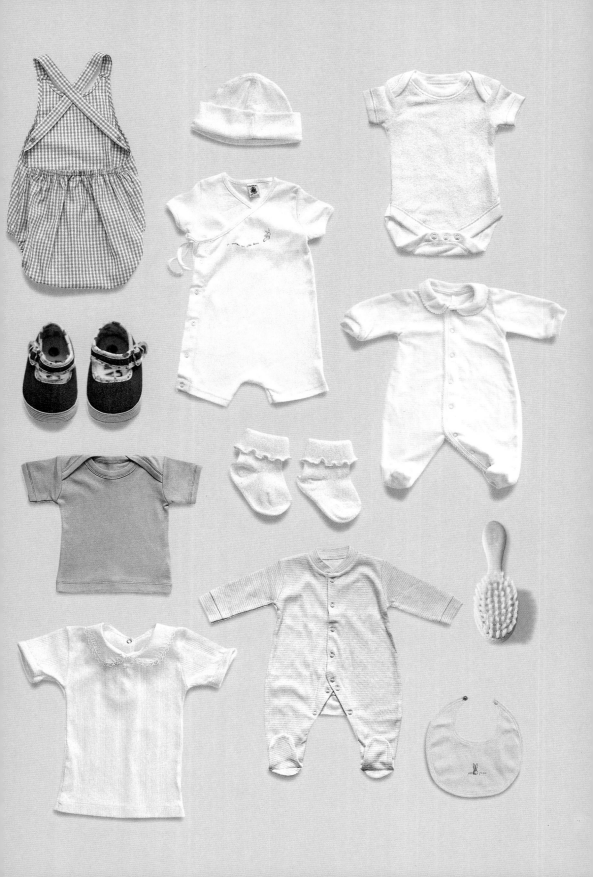

Borrow and return

As babies grow so quickly and their demands are constantly changing, it is a good idea to borrow some of the equipment you will need from friends or family who already have children. This will reduce your costs as well as reduce the clutter in your home as you can return items as soon as your baby has outgrown them. If possible, it's also worth borrowing maternity clothing and books on pregnancy and birth. Just make sure you give the items back in a good condition once you've finished with them, and who knows, maybe you'll be able to return the favor one day!

There are certain items, however, that should be treated with caution. Second-hand items don't always come with the original instruction manuals, and older items may not meet current safety standards. Some items are best bought new for hygiene and safety reasons. Products such as mattresses quickly show signs of wear and tear and can be hard to get clean, so ideally they should not be borrowed. And it is never advisable to borrow (or buy) a second-hand baby car seat, as you need to be certain that it has never been damaged or in a crash. You'll also need the instruction manual, so you can fit and use the seat properly.

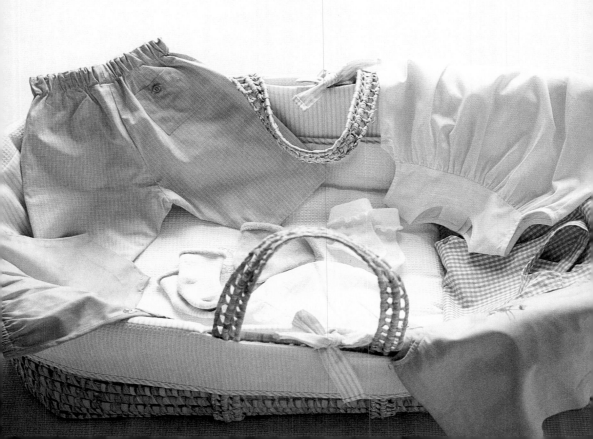

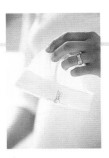

Items I have borrowed

From whom

_____   _____

_____   _____

_____   _____

_____   _____

_____   _____

_____   _____

_____   _____

_____   _____

_____   _____

_____   _____

_____   _____

_____   _____

_____   _____

_____   _____

_____   _____

_____   _____

_____   _____

_____   _____

_____   _____

_____   _____

_____   _____

_____   _____

_____   _____

_____   _____

Notes

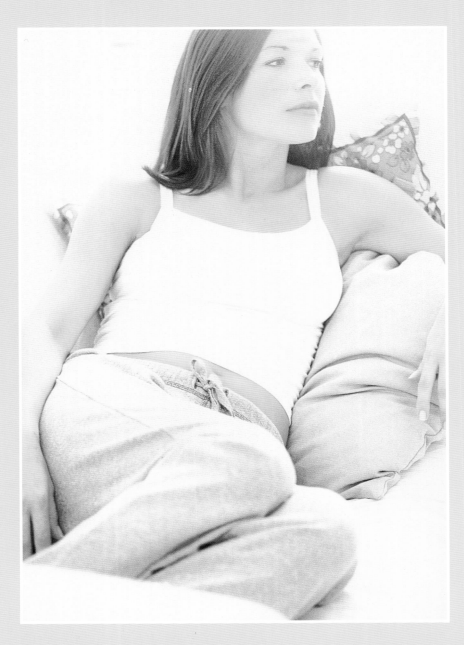

the first trimester

"A journey of a thousand miles must begin with a single step."

The Way of Lao Tzu, Lao Tzu (6th Century BC)

EARLY DAYS

Although you are bound to be excited at the prospect of having a baby, the first three months are also an anxious time in any pregnancy and a time when you are probably trying to keep it a secret from most people. Your body shouldn't change too much over the next 14 weeks but you may be tired and nauseous. You may also be bloated and feel faint.

It's not all bad news though! Just think, this is the start of the most wonderful stage in your life so far, and your body is simply adapting to the task ahead. And in nine months' time you will have a beautiful new baby to love and cherish.

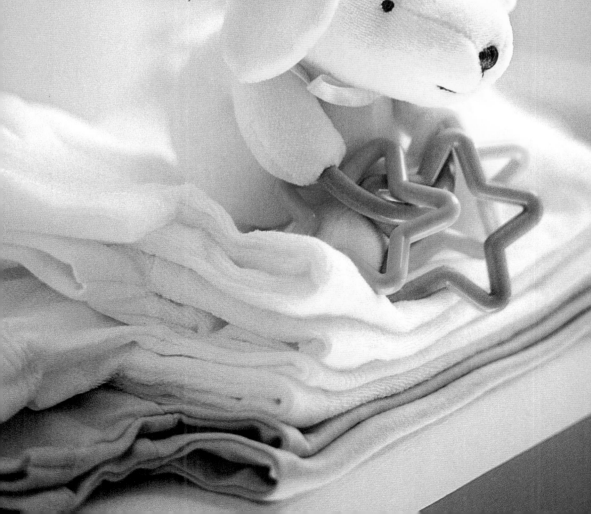

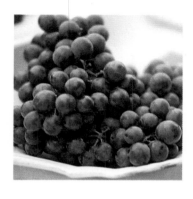

Week 1

To avoid confusion over the exact day your baby is conceived, the first day of pregnancy is taken as the first day of your last period. As today is the first day of your period you won't have conceived yet, but as this is the date your pregnancy will be dated from make a note of it here. Make sure you are eating a well-balanced diet and taking the recommended daily amount of folic acid (400mcg). Avoid taking any drugs or medication that haven't been prescribed for you by your doctor, and, if you are ill, make sure your doctor knows that there is a possibility you could be pregnant before she writes you a prescription.

THINGS TO DO Buy and borrow books on pregnancy. Keep a record of any books you have borrowed on page 63.

Notes
_____
_____
_____
_____
_____
_____
_____
_____
_____
_____
_____
_____
_____
_____
_____
_____
_____

Week 2

As most women ovulate between 12 and 16 days before their next period, ovulation will take place towards the end of this week or the beginning of week 3.

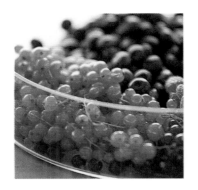

DID YOU KNOW? The sex of your baby is determined by your partner's sperm. However, if you do want to try for a particular sex some schools of thought recommend certain natural ways to increase your chances towards your preferred choice. According to some people it's all in your diet, although you have to keep to the diet for several months before you conceive for it to have an effect. The theory goes that if you want a girl you should eat starchy foods and dairy products, and if it's a boy you're after you should concentrate on meat and fruit. Others say it's all in the timing—and having sex on your ovulation day increases your chances of having a boy. There is some research that disputes this claim, but you could always buy a home ovulation kit and try it out!

Notes

_____

_____

_____

_____

_____

_____

_____

_____

_____

_____

_____

_____

_____

_____

_____

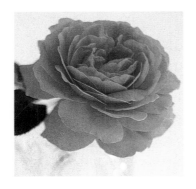

Week 3

You have now conceived! Although some women say they knew they were pregnant from day one, you are unlikely to notice any hormonal changes at this early stage.

How I felt when I found out I was pregnant

_____
_____
_____
_____
_____
_____
_____

How my partner felt

_____
_____
_____
_____
_____
_____
_____

By now you are carrying a tiny cluster of 16 cells, which are the beginnings of your baby. This new life already has a determined sex.

Week 4

You may start to notice some differences at this stage in your pregnancy. Your breasts may be swollen and tender, and you may be feeling quite tired and nauseous.

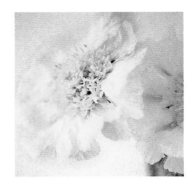

How am I feeling this week?

Energy _Still feeling the same_

Mood _No change_

Appetite _Normal_

Cravings _Greasy food (french fries, cheeseburgers, fried chicken.)_

Sickness _On and of neusea throughout the day._

Notes

Even at this very early stage in your pregnancy your baby's major internal organs are already starting to form.

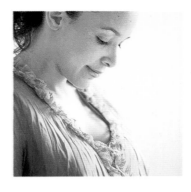

Week 5

By now you will have missed your period and will realize that you are pregnant. There are plenty of reliable home-pregnancy test kits on the market, but it's always a good idea to visit your doctor at this stage. He will be able to tell you the estimated due date (EDD) of your baby and talk through prenatal care and birthing options with you. Start booking some prenatal appointments—you can fill in your appointments on your pregnancy calendar on pages 6—9.

You may want to start thinking about where you want to have your baby—at the hospital or at home. Make a list of the pros and cons for each below.

Hospital birth _____

Home birth _____

Your baby is already changing shape, from a hollow cluster of cells to a long narrow form.

Week 6

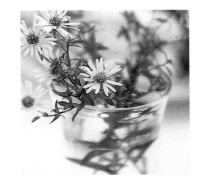

If you decide that you would prefer to give birth in a
hospital and you have a choice of local hospitals, visit the
labor ward of each one before deciding where you want
to have your baby. Find out what facilities they have, what
birthing options they provide—do they have a birthing
pool, for example—and what kind of prenatal care they offer. Also, bear in mind how easy
they are to reach from your home. What are the routes to the hospitals like during rush hour?
What are the parking facilities like? Make a list of your choice of local hospitals below and
note down the pros and cons for each one.

Hospital choices

Pros and cons

By now your growing baby will be about the size of
the very end of your fingertip.

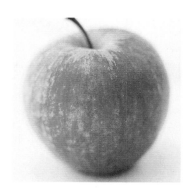

Week 7

By now morning sickness may be a problem. One way to try and keep this under control is to eat little and often—carry snacks like raisins and crackers in your bag just in case you need something when you are out and about.

THINGS TO DO Keep a note here of anything of interest that you read in pregnancy books and magazines.

Notes

The placenta is now starting to form. This will provide your baby with all the nutrients he needs to develop throughout the pregnancy.

Week 8

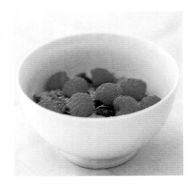

As well as feeling nauseous you may also be feeling very tired and lethargic right now. This is because your heart rate rises and your metabolic rate increases. Try to rest as much as possible, and take comfort in the fact that these feelings—both the tiredness and the nausea—should ease up in the second trimester.

How am I feeling this week?

Energy

_____
_____
_____

Mood

_____
_____
_____

Appetite

_____
_____
_____

Cravings

_____
_____
_____

Sickness

_____
_____

Your baby will now have eyes, although his eyelids will be closed over them. He will also have arms that bend at the elbows, legs that bend at the knees, and his toes will be forming.

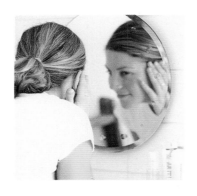

Week 9

Your skin may start to look different now. Pregnancy can cause your skin texture to change so you might need to start using different skin products, especially moisturizers.

How am I feeling this week?

Energy

_____

_____

Mood

_____

Appetite

_____

_____

Cravings

_____

_____

Sickness

_____

_____

Notes

_____

_____

_____

_____

By now the basic structure of all your baby's major organs is in place.

Week 10

By now you may have noticed a change in your body shape—although it certainly won't be dramatic. Try to take regular exercise throughout your pregnancy. Find out if there are any local exercise classes you could attend that are specially tailored for pregnant women. Check at your local swimming pool for classes, for example. Continue to eat healthily during your pregnancy and eat according to your appetite. It is never a good idea to diet during pregnancy, unless advised to do so by your doctor.

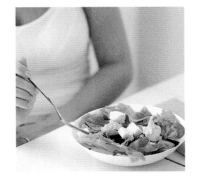

Local exercise class options

_____   _____
_____   _____
_____   _____
_____   _____
_____   _____
_____   _____
_____   _____
_____   _____

Notes

_____
_____
_____
_____
_____

Your baby's weight is now equivalent to that of a large strawberry.

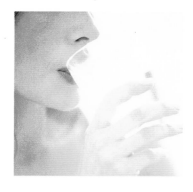

Week 11

You may find that your gums are starting to bleed when you brush your teeth. Visit your dentist for advice on keeping your teeth healthy during your pregnancy. Make sure he knows you are expecting as some treatments, such as X-rays, are not advised during pregnancy.

How am I feeling this week?

Energy

Mood

Appetite

Cravings

Sickness

Notes

Your baby is now beginning to suck, swallow, and yawn.

Week 12

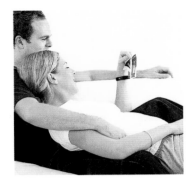

At some point around now you may be offered a 'dating' ultrasound scan, especially if there is some question about the gestational age of your baby. This will be a very exciting experience as it will be the first time you and your partner will see your baby. You may also be offered a nuchal translucency scan at any time between 11 to 14 weeks to screen for Down's Syndrome and other chromosomal disorders as well as congenital heart problems.

How did I feel before having the scan?

_____

_____

_____

How did I feel when I saw the scan?

_____

_____

_____

_____

How did my partner feel?

_____

_____

_____

At just 12 weeks all the major organs are fully formed, although your baby is still only about 2½in (6cm) long.

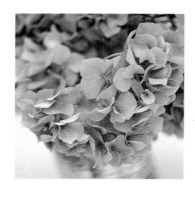

Week 13

THINGS TO DO From now on your body will begin changing quite dramatically as your baby grows in size. You might like to keep a week-by-week photographic record of your changing body shape. The easiest way to do this is to ask your partner or a friend to take profile shots of you using your smartphone or a digital camera. The series of photographs that result will be a fascinating record to look back on in the years to come.

How am I feeling this week?

Energy

Mood

Appetite

Cravings

Sickness

Notes

Your baby now weighs approximately one ounce and is about the size of a peach. If she is a girl, her ovaries will now contain all the eggs she'll ever have.

Week 14

Now that your pregnancy is beginning to show, you might want to start sharing your exciting news with your friends and family. Make a list below of all the people you would like to tell.

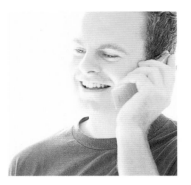

Who we need tell	Their reaction

At this stage your baby's toenails and fingernails will start developing.

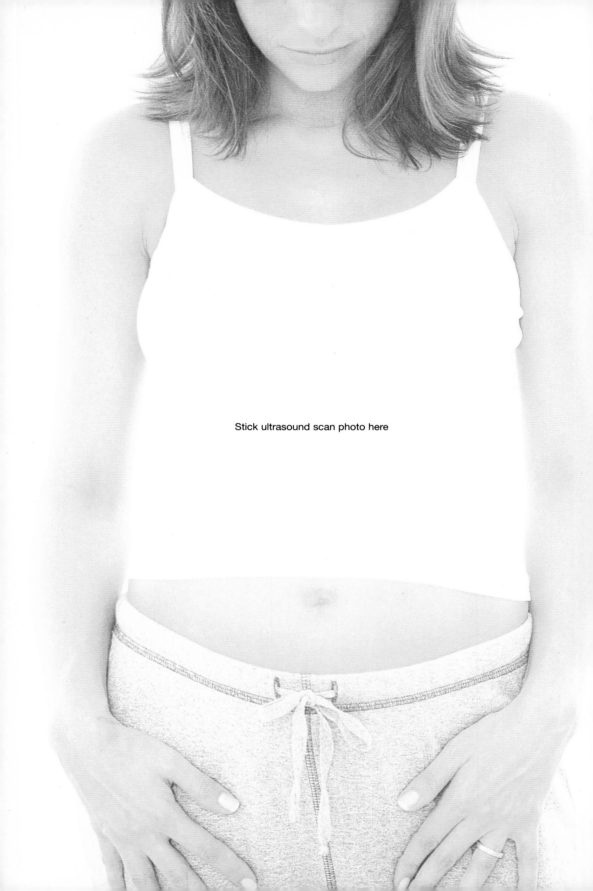

Stick ultrasound scan photo here

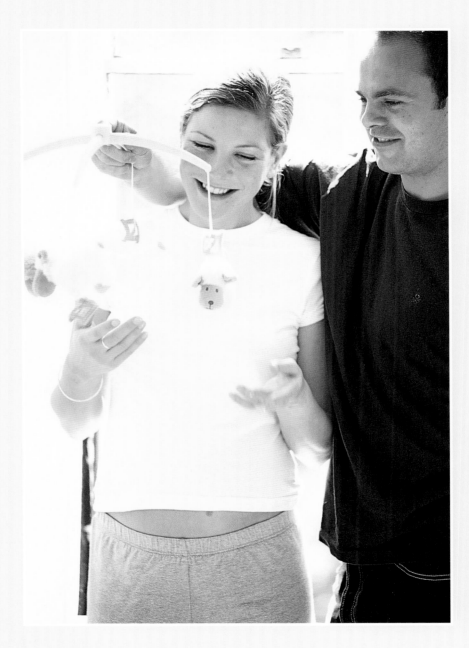

the second trimester

NEARLY HALFWAY THERE

Now you've reached the second trimester. This will probably be the most enjoyable part of your pregnancy. Your energy should return, the morning sickness should ease off, and you are not yet large enough to find the extra weight a major burden. Take advantage of your new-found energy to go out with friends, spend time with your partner, and generally have some fun.

This is also an exciting time as your bump will really start to develop—and around 18—20 weeks you will start to feel your baby moving around. Be sure to record the first time you feel him kick, not forgetting the first time you get offered a seat on the bus or train!

"A baby is an inestimable blessing."

Mark Twain (1835—1910)

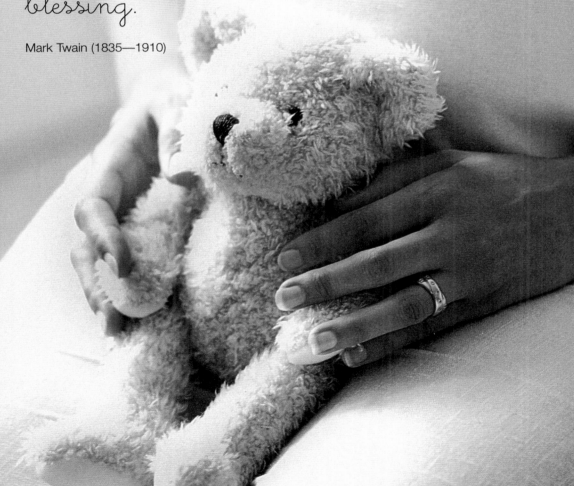

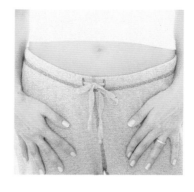

Week 15

Your sickness may have completely eased off by now, although with your expanding waistline you're probably having trouble getting into some of your clothes. If you don't like the idea of wearing maternity clothes, choose items that are a couple of sizes larger than usual.

Elasticated and drawstring trousers are a good option and should last you for a few weeks. You only need a few basic items but don't buy everything at once as at this stage it will be hard to tell what is going to happen to your body shape. See if you can borrow any maternity clothes from friends or family who have had children.

What clothes have I borrowed?

From whom

Your baby will now fit into the palm of your hand.

Week 16

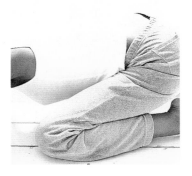

If you haven't done so already, check out what birthing or parenting classes are available to you. Make a list and then work out which ones you would like to sign up for. You can keep notes of what you learn at the classes on pages 41—45.

Birthing and parenting classes
_____
_____
_____
_____
_____
_____
_____
_____
_____
_____

How am I feeling this week?

Energy
_____

Mood
_____

Appetite
_____

Cravings
_____

Sickness
_____
_____

By now your baby is very active and can suck her thumb and make a fist.

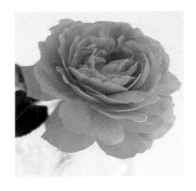

Week 17

A dark line may appear down the center of your abdomen at this stage in your pregnancy; this is called the linea nigra. It marks the division of your abdominal muscles, which separate slightly in order to make room for your expanding uterus.

THINGS TO DO Continue keeping a photographic record of your changing body shape—the changes are going to be much more dramatic from now on as your bump continues to grow.

How am I feeling this week?

Energy

Mood

Appetite

Cravings

Sickness

This is probably the earliest that you will be able to feel your baby's movements, but don't worry if you can't feel him yet—it can happen later in the trimester, especially if you're a first-time mother.

Week 18

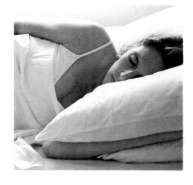

You may have started having quite vivid dreams, although this may occur later in pregnancy for some women. Try to remember them when you wake up and write them down in a dream diary or just jot them down in your journal notes—it will make for interesting reading later on.

DID YOU KNOW? When your baby is born he will have 300 bones in his body. However, as he grows up some of them will fuse together so by the time he reaches adulthood he will have just 206 bones.

Notes

_____

_____

_____

_____

_____

_____

_____

_____

_____

_____

_____

Your baby's eyes are now sensitive to light and his eye muscles are strong enough to move them from side to side while looking down. He will also be able to hear loud noises, though he will be unable to interpret them until the third trimester.

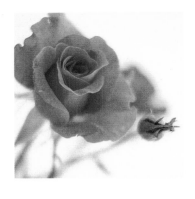

Week 19

You may be having your fetal anomaly ultrasound scan some time between 18 and 22 weeks. This is a serious diagnostic tool that enables the ultrasound technician to check for any development or growth problems your baby may be experiencing. The technician may also be able to tell you your baby's sex at this stage, should you wish to know. It is worth discussing with your partner now whether you want to know this.

Do we want to know our baby's sex?

Pros	Cons

How am I feeling this week?

Energy

Mood

Appetite

Cravings

Sickness

Your baby's head is now about one third of the size of her body.

Week 20

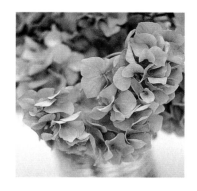

Before you go for the fetal anomaly ultrasound scan, talk to your doctor about exactly what the scan will be checking, and how accurate the measurements are. Make a note of any anxieties or questions you have about the results of the scan, and possible consequences for you and your baby.

Questions I would like to ask when I attend the scan:

At 20 weeks your baby's first teeth will have developed in her gums.

Week 21

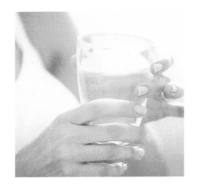

Your weight will have been gradually increasing throughout your pregnancy and you will have been gaining weight steadily from about week 12, but most weight is gained after week 20. Weight gain in pregnancy does vary, depending on a woman's BMI before she became pregnant, but The Institute of Medicine recommends that most expectant moms of a normal weight (a BMI of 18.5–24.9) gain between 25–35 pounds during their pregnancy. If you are underweight, you should gain 28 to 40 pounds, while overweight women should only gain 15 to 25 pounds. Although your appetite may also be increasing, you don't need to eat for two—your body only needs approximately an additional 200 calories a day. You should never diet during pregnancy, except under doctor's orders.

How am I feeling this week?

Energy

Mood

Appetite

Cravings

Sickness

Your baby's fingers are now fully formed and have the ability to grasp.

Week 22

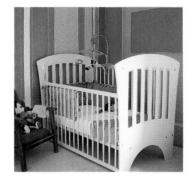

How exciting—you are now over halfway there! This is a good time to start thinking about decorating the nursery—although if there's any painting to be done get your partner to do it as the fumes might make you feel sick or give you a headache. If you have found out the sex of your baby you may want to choose the traditional pink for a girl and blue for a boy. If you don't know what sex your baby is, you may want to decorate your baby's bedroom in a neutral colour. Turn to page 56 to make a note of your ideas about decorating the nursery.

Notes

_____

_____

_____

_____

_____

_____

_____

_____

_____

_____

_____

_____

_____

_____

_____

Your baby's hearing will now be acute and, although sounds will be muffled by the amniotic fluid, loud noises could make him jump.

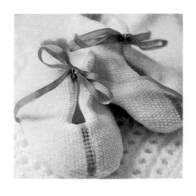

Week 23

Due to the hormonal changes you are experiencing, you may be having problems with your eyes—for example your contact lenses may be more uncomfortable than usual. These problems are only temporary, but if you do wear glasses visit your eye doctor for a check-up.

How am I feeling this week?

Energy

Mood

Appetite

Cravings

Sickness

This week your baby's eyelids will open, although she won't be able to see much because the womb is dark—it will get lighter as the skin stretches—and her visual range is limited until a few weeks after birth.

Week 24

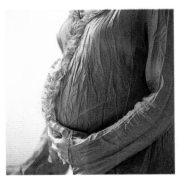

Your energy levels should have risen considerably so it would be a good time to do some shopping in preparation for your new arrival or to catch up with friends. By now, your baby's nervous system and muscles will have developed enough to enable her to move around inside you. The first time you feel her making small movements will be an exhilarating experience. Make a note below of how it feels.

What does it feel like?

_____

_____

_____

_____

Do you like the sensation?

_____

_____

_____

_____

Does the baby stop kicking when your partner touches your tummy?

_____

_____

_____

With the exception of the lungs, all your baby's major organs are now functioning. All the facial features are formed too, so at this stage she will look very much like she will at birth, only smaller.

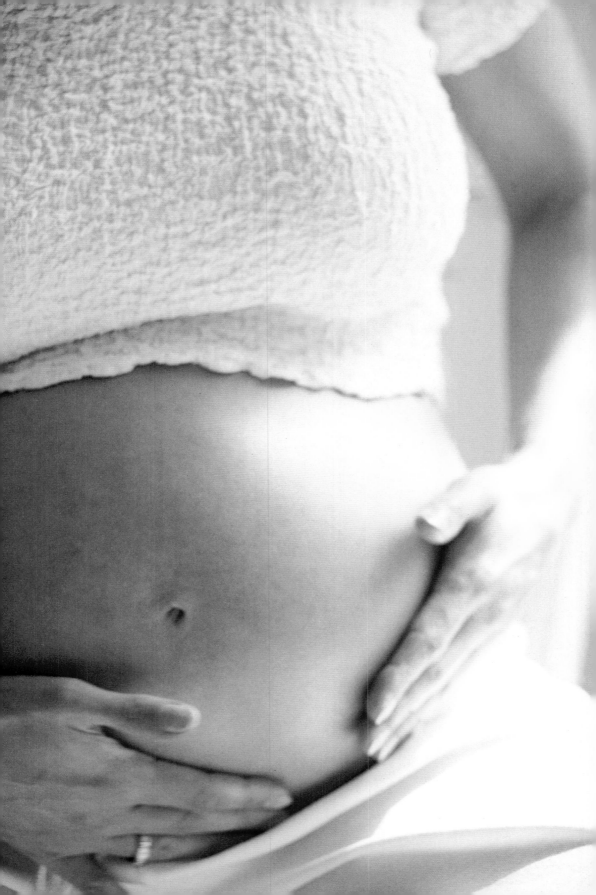

Week 25

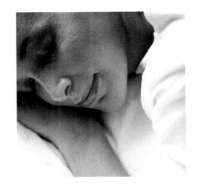

If you would like one last trip before you've got your hands full, your second trimester is the time to do it. You have higher energy levels than you've had in a while, you won't be too large and cumbersome yet and, most importantly, the airlines are still willing to let you on board!

After 28 weeks, you may need need a signed letter from your doctor confirming your due date and that you are safe to fly. If you have had a normal, healthy pregnancy, most airlines will allow you to travel up until 36 weeks pregnant (32 weeks for twins). Check with specific carriers for airline regulations and always ask about any restrictions before you book a ticket. Make sure that you're covered by your travel insurance too, as many policies aren't valid for women in the late stages of pregnancy.

How am I feeling this week?

Energy

Mood

Appetite

Cravings

Sickness

By now your baby's cells that promote conscious thought are developing.

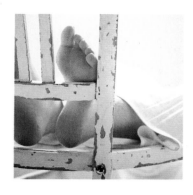

Week 26

Increased movements from your baby may be stopping you from sleeping properly at night, especially as in many cases a baby is much more active at night time. Make sure you grab some sleep whenever you can, as you should try to get plenty of rest.

THINGS TO DO Make sure you do your pelvic floor exercises regularly. This will help prevent stress incontinence during pregnancy and once your baby is born.

How am I feeling this week?

Energy

Mood

Appetite

Cravings

Sickness

Notes

Your baby's nostrils have started to open and he will make breathing movements in preparation for when he will have to draw air after the birth.

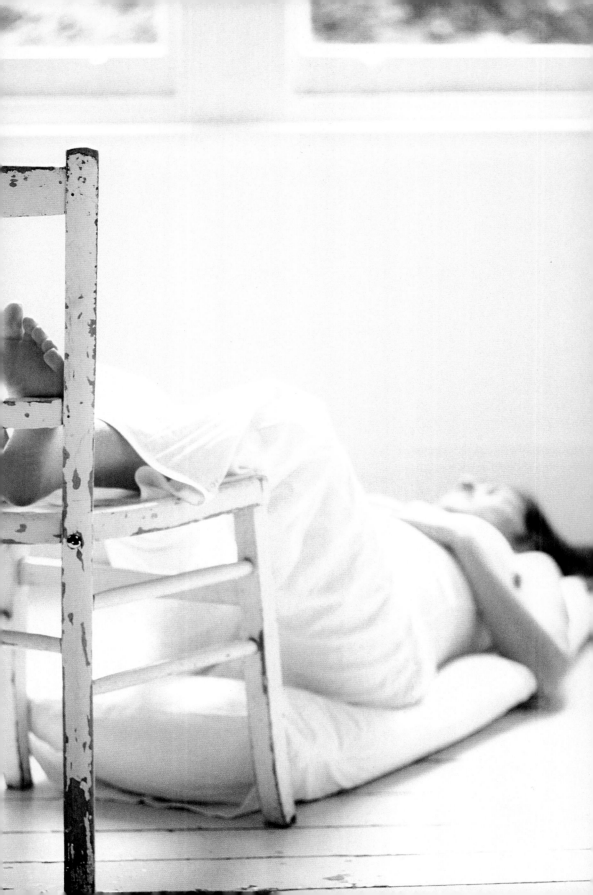

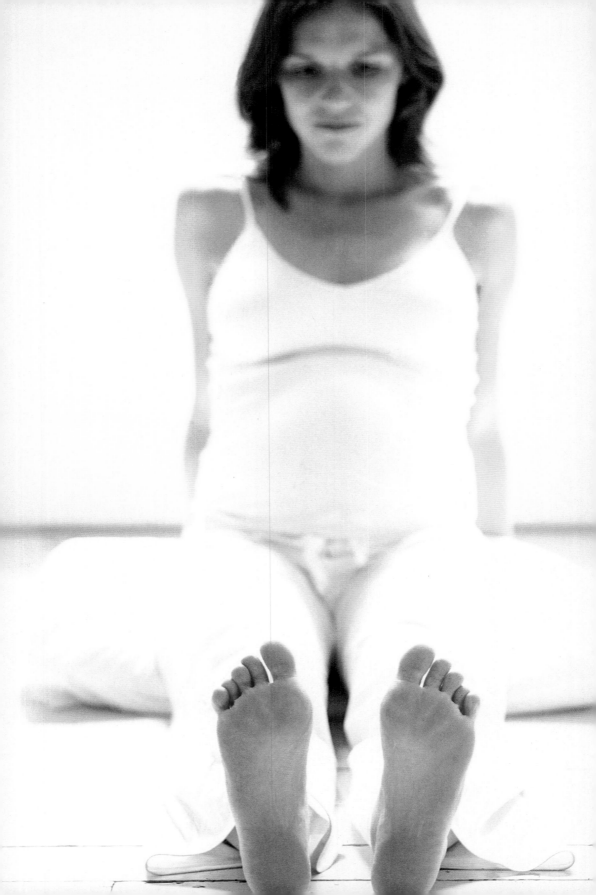

Week 27

As your bump becomes more pronounced you may be getting increasingly bad backache. There are several things you can try to reduce its severity.

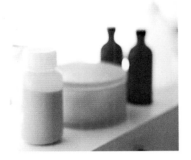

• Keep an eye on your posture. Despite the amount of weight you are carrying out front, don't be tempted to arch your back and don't slouch—this will only make it worse.
• Get your partner to give you a back rub or massage using a few drops of essential oil mixed with a carrier oil. Essential oils that are recommended for use in pregnancy include: camomile, citrus, geranium and lavender. There is a long list of essential oils that should be avoided in pregnancy. If you are not sure whether an oil is safe for you to use, check first with your doctor.
• Avoiding lifting any heavy weights if you can. If you do need to lift something from the floor, bend your knees keeping your back as straight as you can. Lift the object by straightening your legs so that your leg muscles do the work, not your back.
• If the pain is really bad consult your doctor.

How am I feeling this week?

Energy

Mood

Appetite

Cravings

Sickness

Although she is growing rapidly, your baby still only weighs just over two pounds—about the same weight as a small bag of sugar.

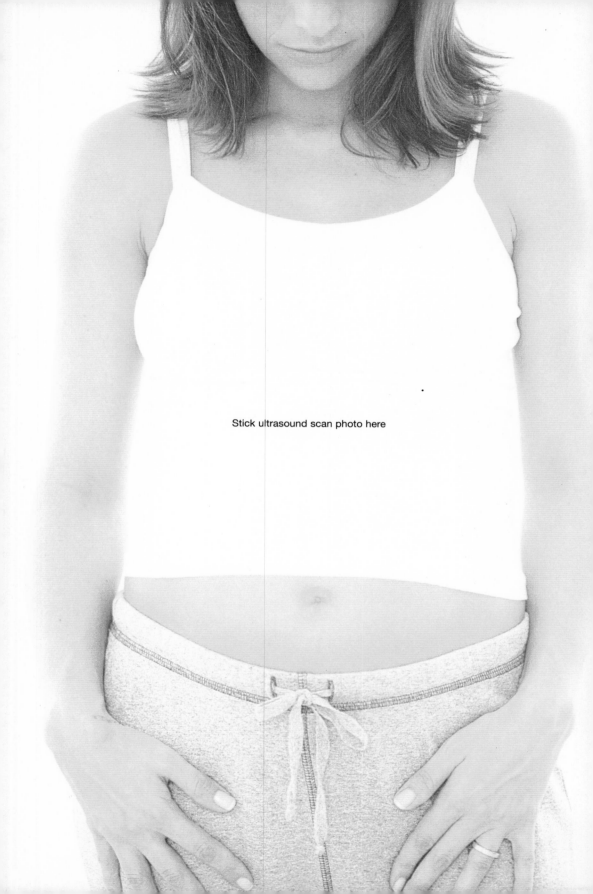

Stick ultrasound scan photo here

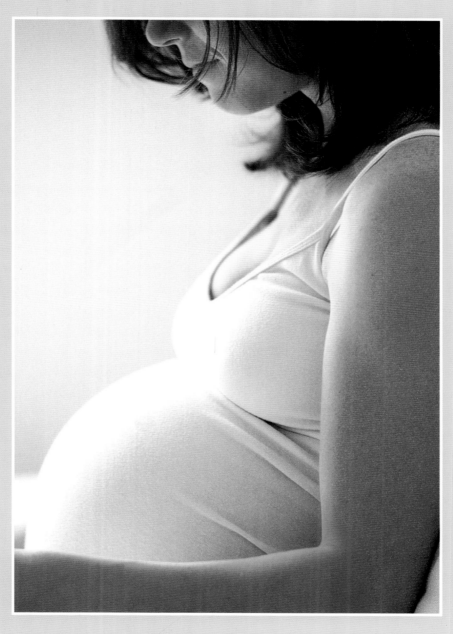

the third trimester

"The most effective kind of education is that a child should play amongst lovely things."

Plato (c. 429—347 BC)

THE HOME STRETCH

You're into the third trimester and well over halfway through your pregnancy. You may start feeling like you've been pregnant forever—indeed you probably can't remember life before pregnancy! The sheer size of your stomach will make it hard for you do things towards the end of this trimester—making you short of breath, tired, and preventing you from getting a good night's sleep. Grab naps where and when you can.

It's time to make sure you, your partner, and your home are ready for the new arrival. Preparing for your baby as much as possible now will stop you worrying about not being ready for him when he is finally born. Spend time going to baby shops with your partner and choose a special toy to welcome your baby into the world.

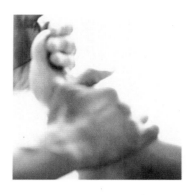

Week 28

You are now on the home straight—the third trimester—and you should be feeling fantastic, but take care not to overdo it. Spend some time every day relaxing with your feet up. This will help to relieve any stress and make you less likely to suffer from swollen feet and ankles—a common complaint during pregnancy. Your hair should look and feel thicker and healthier—now is a good time to go to the hairdresser's and get an easy-to-manage hairstyle.

How am I feeling this week?

Energy

Mood

Appetite

Cravings

Sickness

Notes

Your baby is now aware of some external light.

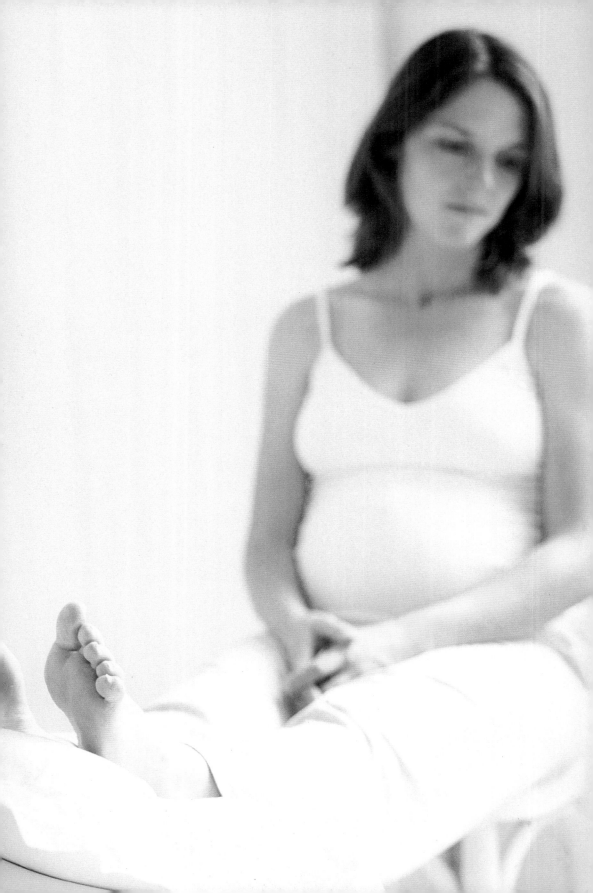

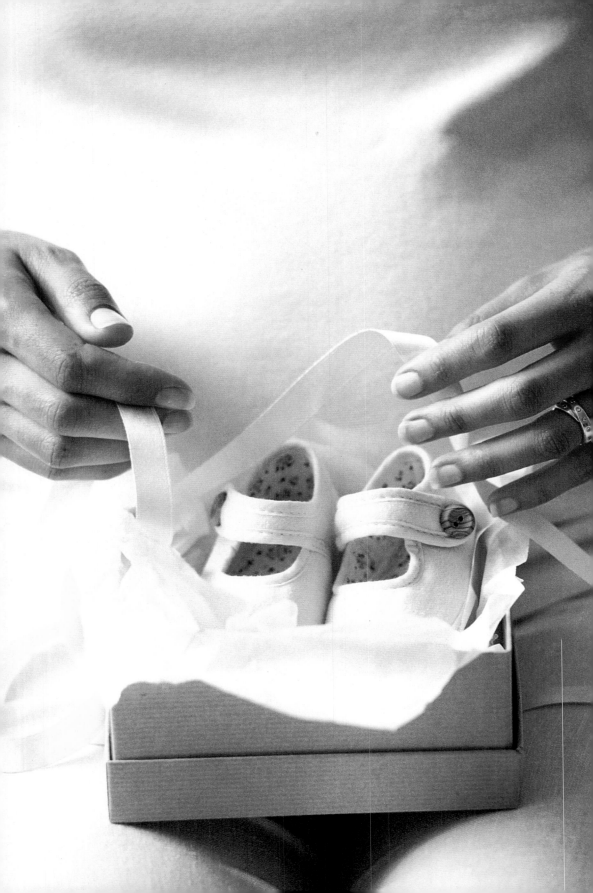

Week 29

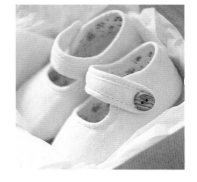

As you enter your third trimester, make sure you have planned your maternity leave. If you are planning to take unpaid family leave, you must provide your employer with at least 30 days' notice of your intentions. Even if you are working right up to your due date, it's important to have everything arranged with your employer as early as possible, as maternity rights are the last thing you want to worry about once you go on your maternity leave.

How am I feeling this week?

Energy

Mood

Appetite

Cravings

Sickness

Notes

Your baby now has eyelashes on her eyelids.

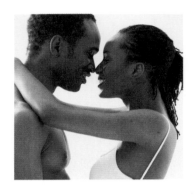

Week 30

By this stage you probably have the impression you've been pregnant forever and may be feeling a bit fed up. Make sure you talk to your partner about how you're feeling so you don't end up arguing over petty things.

THINGS TO DO Start thinking about what you want to include in your birth plan. Discuss your options with your friends from birthing classes and people you know who have already had children. Fill in your preferences on page 139.

How am I feeling this week?

Energy

Mood

Appetite

Cravings

Sickness

Notes

Your baby is peeing a pint of urine a day, which your kidneys are recycling!

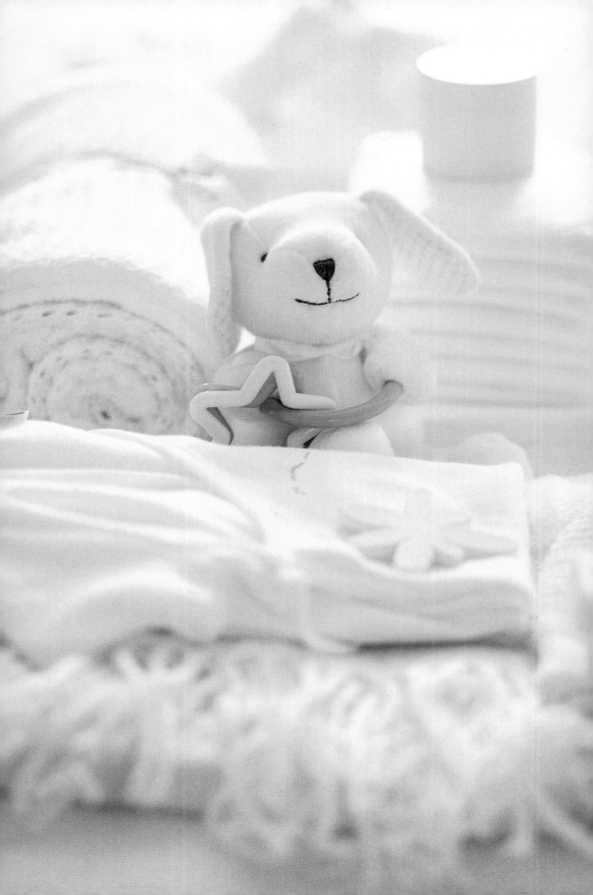

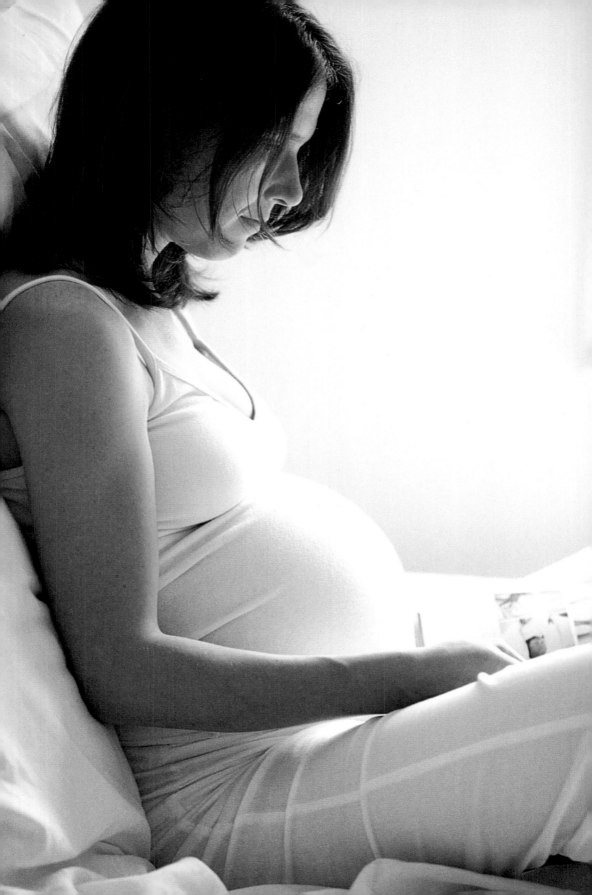

Week 31

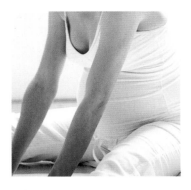

You may be suffering from cramps in your calf—especially during the night. There are a number of ways you can try to prevent this from happening. However if symptoms continue consult your doctor or midwife.

- Avoid wearing heels. Wearing flat shoes will stop your calf muscles getting bunched up.
- Relieve cramp by gently massaging the affected area.
- Stretch the muscle by flexing your foot and pushing into your heel.
- Cramp can be caused by mineral imbalances so if you are short of any you should increase your intake. But check with your doctor before you start taking supplements.

How am I feeling this week?

Energy

Mood

Appetite

Cravings

Sickness

Your baby's growth will start to slow down between now and his birth.

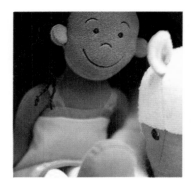

Week 32

You may be feeling practice contractions—called Braxton Hicks contractions. Most women experience these during the last few months of pregnancy. You will feel your stomach tighten for about 30 seconds and this can happen a few times a day. These contractions mean your uterus is practicing for the strong contractions needed in labor, but don't worry, they don't mean you are about to go into real labor.

THINGS TO DO If you haven't done so already, start thinking about ordering some of the items you will need as soon as your baby arrives. Some larger products, such as cribs and carriages, may take up to six weeks to be delivered.

How am I feeling this week?

Energy

Mood

Appetite

Cravings

Sickness

By now your baby's lungs will have developed most of their airways and airsacs ready to use after birth.

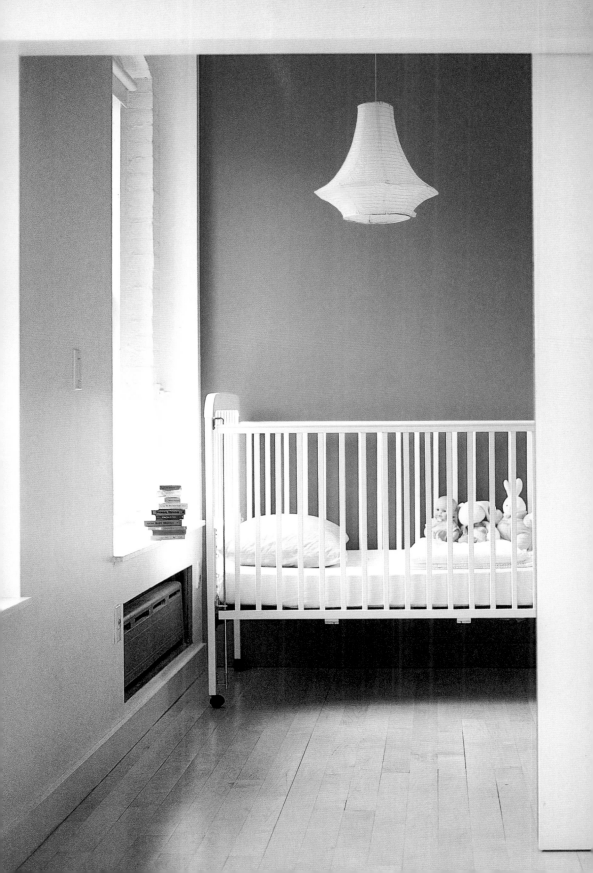

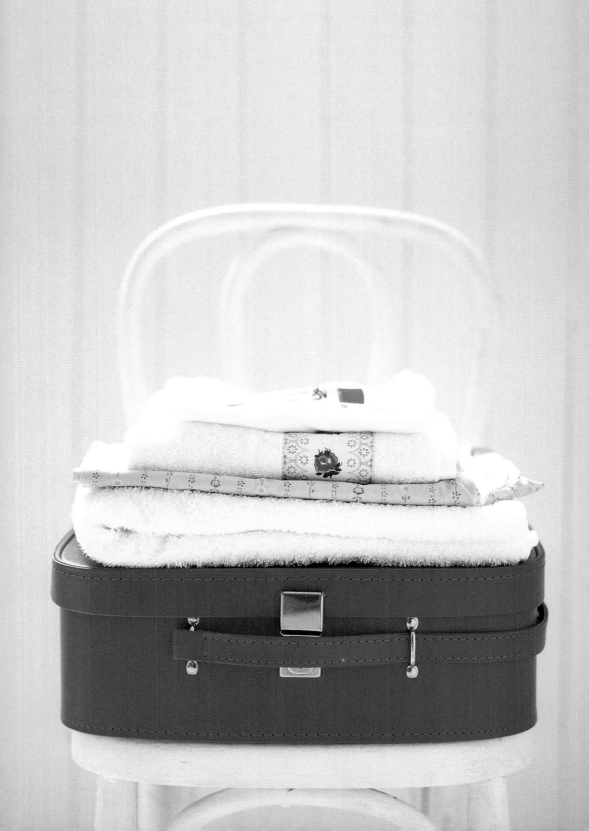

Week 33

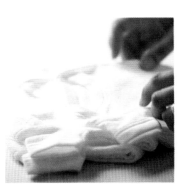

As your baby moves you will sometimes be able to see the outline of a little fist or foot in your abdomen. Share such experiences with your partner so he feels as involved in your baby's development as you are.

THINGS TO DO This is a good time to pack your hospital bag (see page 140 for a checklist of things to pack). If you have opted for a home birth sort out all the things you will need to have at home ready for when you go into labor.

How am I feeling this week?

Energy
_____
_____

Mood
_____
_____

Appetite
_____
_____

Cravings
_____
_____

Sickness
_____
_____

Notes
_____
_____
_____

Your baby's chest movements may cause her to hiccup occasionally. You will feel these as regular little jumps.

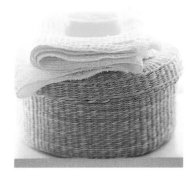

Week 34

For a few women the dreaded morning sickness may return at this late stage in pregnancy. If there has been any concern about the position or size of your baby, your practictioner may schedule an additional ultrasound scan around this time to check that all is well.

How am I feeling this week?

Energy

Mood

Appetite

Cravings

Sickness

Notes

By this time your baby may well be positioned with his head down so he's in the right position ready for his birth.

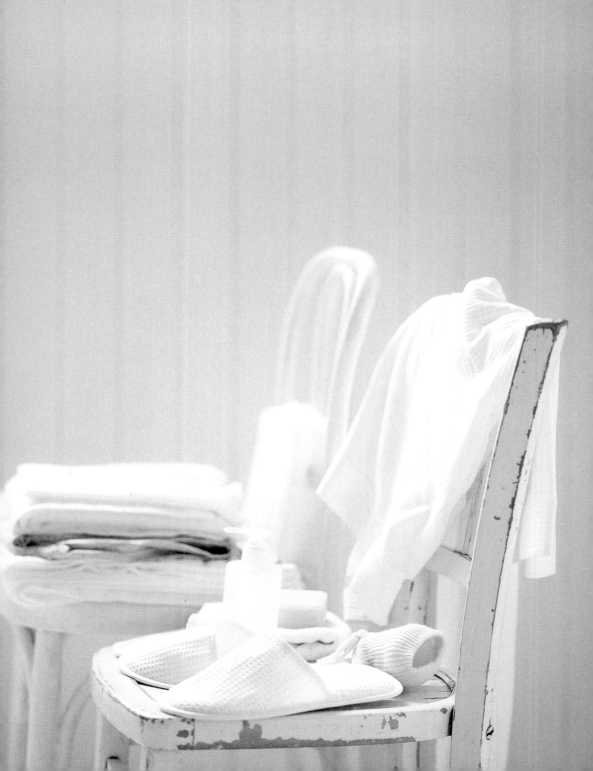

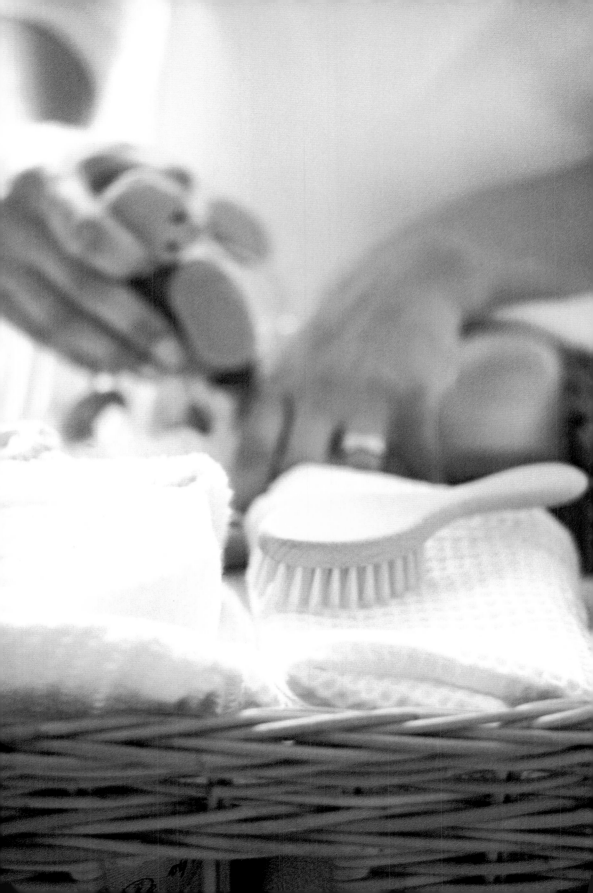

Week 35

Your size, discomfort, and overall pregnant feeling may be making you feel less than attractive. Make sure you take time to let your partner know how you feel so he can reassure you.

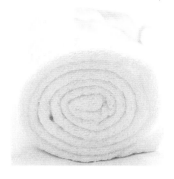

THINGS TO DO Make a list of all the people you will want to inform once your new arrival is here. Things are likely to be pretty hectic once your baby is born, so it might be a good idea to write out or print off some name and address labels in preparation for the announcements.

How am I feeling this week?

Energy

Mood

Appetite

Cravings

Sickness

Your baby is starting to run out of room now. If her squirming is bothering you, try having a long bath to make yourself more comfortable.

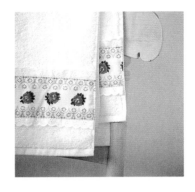

Week 36

You've probably stopped working by now and are relaxing at home. Spend lots of time pampering yourself, so you are as relaxed as possible when D-day arrives. This is also a good time to buy any last-minute items you think you might need for the birth or the nursery.

How am I feeling this week?

Energy

Mood

Appetite

Cravings

Sickness

Notes

At this point your baby's fingernails and toenails are fully grown.

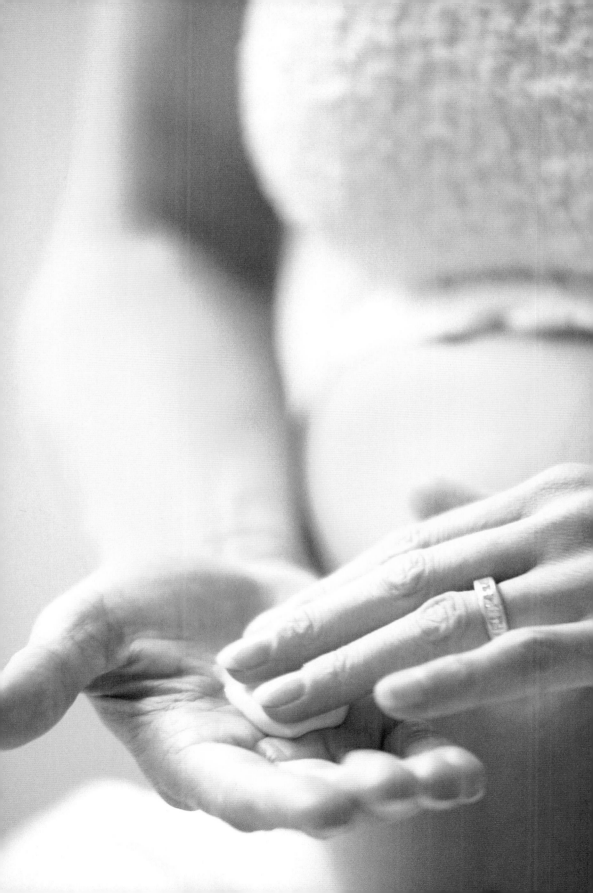

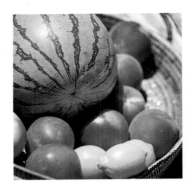

Week 37

You are nearly there! However, 95 percent of healthy babies are born on days other than their due date—generally within two weeks of the estimated date—so get ready, he could be coming any time now.

THINGS TO DO Make sure you have a fully stocked pantry and freezer. Buy ready-meals, rice, pasta, canned food, long life milk, and other foodstuff that will last—supermarket shopping will be the last thing you and your partner want to do once you bring your precious bundle home. Make a list of all the essentials on the opposite page.

How am I feeling this week?

Energy

Mood

Appetite

Cravings

Sickness

Notes

Your baby's head may drop down into your pelvis now, ready for action, but there's still plenty of time.

Shopping list

_____ _____
_____ _____
_____ _____
_____ _____
_____ _____
_____ _____
_____ _____
_____ _____
_____ _____
_____ _____
_____ _____
_____ _____
_____ _____
_____ _____
_____ _____
_____ _____
_____ _____
_____ _____
_____ _____
_____ _____
_____ _____
_____ _____

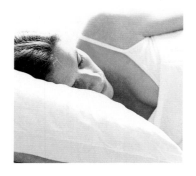

Week 38

Hopefully you will start finding it easier to breathe now if your baby has dropped lower into your pelvis. But the need to urinate frequently may be back with a vengeance!

How am I feeling this week?

Energy

Mood

Appetite

Cravings

Sickness

Notes

Your baby is now a good size and weight. She is ready to be born.

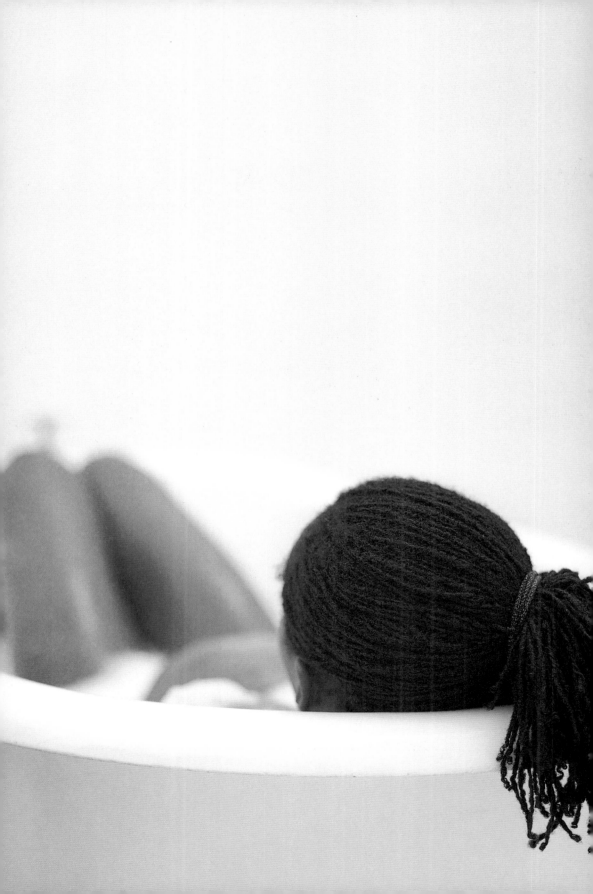

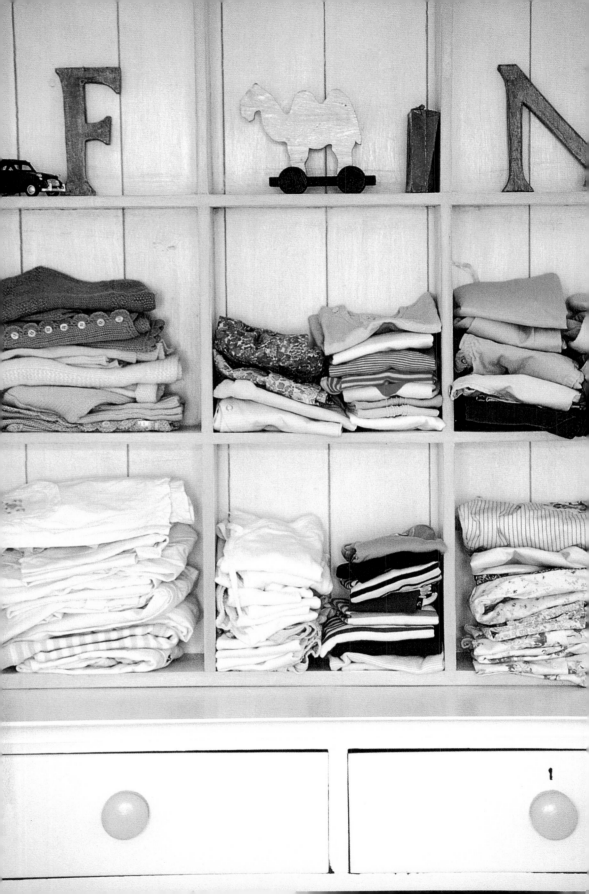

Week 39

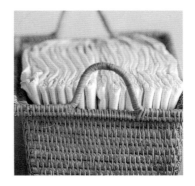

You're probably starting to feel really fed up and to think you've been pregnant forever. Hang on in there—you haven't got long to go now. You may notice a sudden urge to clean and tidy your home. This is your nesting instinct coming into play, you want to make sure everything is ready for the baby's arrival. Don't overdo it.

How am I feeling this week?

Energy

Mood

Appetite

Cravings

Sickness

Notes

The bones in your baby's skull are able to slide over each other and overlap so his head can pass through the birth canal without being damaged.

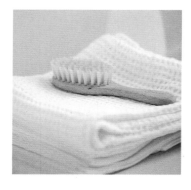

Week 40

After a nine-month wait, your due week has finally arrived! However, as only five percent of babies are actually born on their due date, don't be surprised if yours doesn't stick to the schedule!

How am I feeling this week?

Energy

Mood

Appetite

Cravings

Sickness

Notes

A baby has no functioning tear ducts for the first couple of weeks—during this time her first cries will be tearless ones.

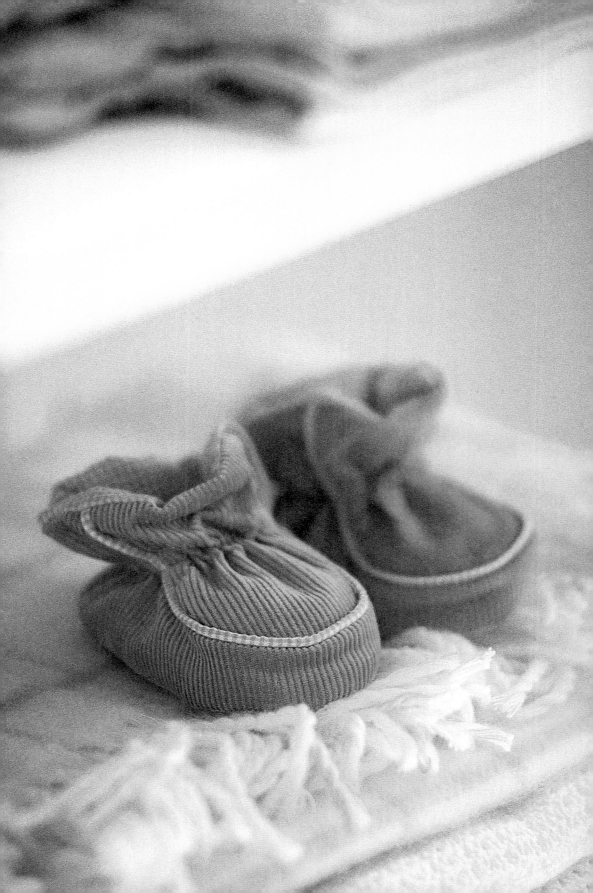

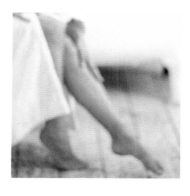

Week 41

You're now overdue, but try not to feel impatient—this is quite common, especially for a first-time mom. Use the extra time to relax, watch television, read a book, catch up with friends, and generally look after yourself. If your cellphone constantly rings with family and friends eager to find out if you've given birth yet, it might be a good idea to screen your calls or update your voicemail message or Facebook page with a status report every day, so you don't get too frustrated with answering the phone and saying the same thing over and over!

How do I feel now I'm overdue?

_____

_____

_____

_____

_____

_____

_____

How am I feeling this week?

Energy

_____

Mood

_____

Appetite

_____

Cravings

_____

Sickness

_____

Week 42

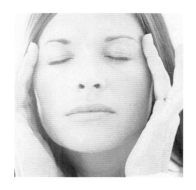

The end is in sight—your baby is likely to be born this week. Read up about being induced so you are prepared for this should your baby still not want to come out of his own accord.

How do I feel now I am still overdue?

_____

_____

_____

_____

_____

_____

_____

_____

_____

_____

How am I feeling this week?

Energy

_____

Mood

_____

Appetite

_____

Cravings

_____

Sickness

_____

Stick our first photo of mom and/or dad and baby here

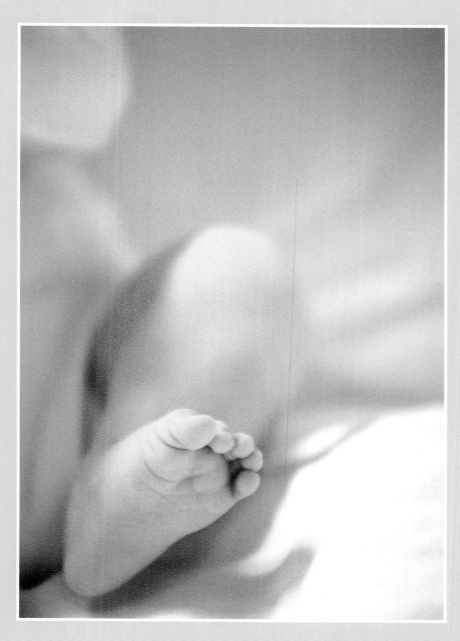

the labor and birth

"Our birth is but a sleep and a forgetting."

Intimations of Immortality, William Wordsworth (1770—1850)

COUNTDOWN TO D-DAY

As your due date approaches you are bound to start focusing more and more on the actual birth itself. The anticipation both you and your partner may feel before this massive event is almost incomparable to anything else you will experience in life—particularly if this is your first pregnancy. Make sure you are well prepared and have read through and discussed all of your birthing options thoroughly. You and your partner should discuss with each other and with your midwife any anxieties you have.

Remember it is you who will be going through the labour and for the most part you can control what happens to you and when. You can determine what pain relief you want (or don't want), what position you want to give birth in and you can even choose what music you want to listen to—this is the one time you will get away with listening to your Carpenters CD!

My thoughts about the birth

I feel: _____

_____

_____

I am worried about: _____

_____

_____

My partner feels: _____

_____

_____

My partner is worried about: _____

_____

_____

Writing a birth plan

When drawing up your birth plan make sure you are familiar with all your options and base your final decisions on what you really want. It's a good idea to discuss this with your midwife and other mothers or mothers-to-be as they may have thought about something that hasn't occurred to you, but try to keep an open mind in case things don't go according to plan. Here are just a few questions you might want to consider before putting pen to paper.

How do you feel about being induced, should you go past your due date?

Who do you want to be present at the birth?

Do you want your partner to be present at all times?

Do you plan to have a doula attend the birth?

Do you want music played or the lights dimmed while you're in labor?

Do you want your medical team to offer you pain relief, or would you rather they waited for you to ask for it?

What are your preferred methods of pain relief?

Are there any types of pain relief you would like to avoid?

Do you want to be as active as possible during labor?

What position would you prefer to give birth in?

Would you prefer to have an episiotomy or wait to see if you tear naturally?

Do you want to see your baby's head being delivered?

Do you want your baby delivered straight to your abdomen?

Would you like to hold baby straight after delivery?

Who do you want to cut the umbilical cord?

Do you plan to bank or donate the cord blood?

Do you want a midwife or a lactation consultant to help you breastfeed?

Would you like your labor partner to be present if you have to have a C-section?

Do you want to deliver the placenta spontaneously and without assistance?

After birth, would you and your partner like to be left alone with your baby?

My birth plan

_____

_____

_____

_____

_____

_____

_____

_____

_____

_____

_____

_____

_____

_____

_____

_____

_____

_____

_____

_____

_____

_____

_____

_____

_____

_____

_____

_____

_____

My hospital bag checklist

For me:

Birth plan

Old T-shirt/nightdress for birth

Socks

Slippers

Water spray (to cool me down)

Mirror (if I want to see the baby being born)

Wash cloths and towels

Camera/video

Toiletries

Tissues

Hot water bottle

Snacks for me/my partner

Music/magazines/playing cards

Coins for pay phone

Front-opening nightdress

Dressing gown

2—3 maternity/nursing bras

Disposable underwear

Maternity sanitary towels

Breast pads

Coming home clothes

Extra items

For baby:

2—3 sleepsuits

2—3 T-shirts

Blanket

Hat

Diapers

Cotton balls

Cream—diaper ointment/Vaseline

Car seat

Extra items

Additional items needed for a home birth:

Pillows or large cushions

Lamp or flashlight

Clean sheets

Plastic sheeting

Hot water and soap

Garbage bags

Extra items

Record of my labor

My labor started at _____ on _____

I went into the hospital at _____ on _____

I went to the hospital by _____

_____

When I arrived at the hospital I _____

_____

_____

_____

_____

_____

_____

How I felt at this stage _____

_____

_____

_____

_____

_____

_____

_____

_____

My baby was delivered at _____ on _____

I was in labor for _____ hours _____ minutes

What pain relief did I use?

_____

_____

_____

_____

_____

Who was present at the birth?

_____

_____

_____

Who cut the baby's umbilical cord?

_____

_____

Did the baby cry right away?

_____

_____

Was childbirth how I imagined it to be?

_____

_____

_____

_____

_____

_____

_____

_____

_____

_____

In what ways was it different?

_____

_____

_____

_____

_____

If I did it all over again would I change anything?

_____

_____

_____

_____

_____

_____

How do I feel now our baby is born?

_____

_____

_____

_____

How does my partner feel now our baby is born?

_____

_____

_____

_____

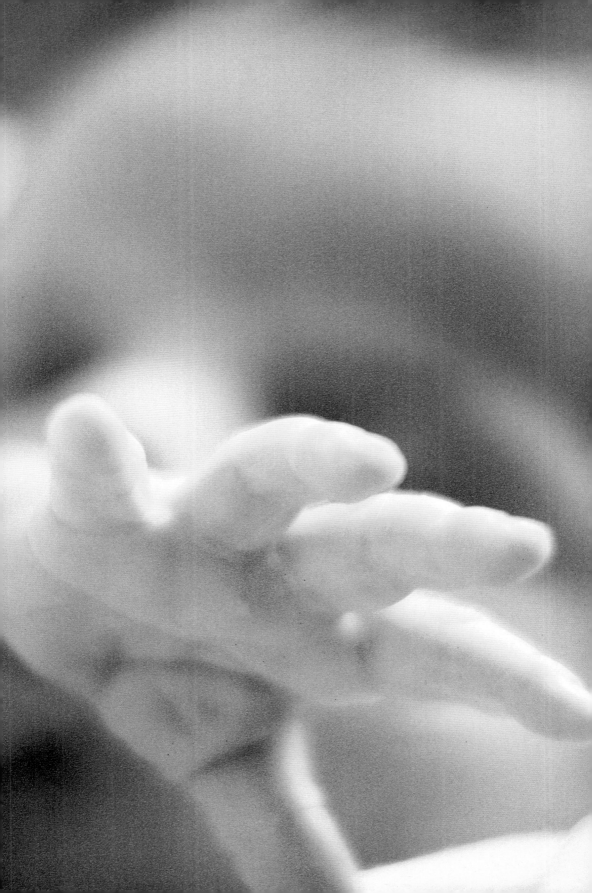

The people we need to call after the birth

Name   Telephone number

_____   _____

_____   _____

_____   _____

_____   _____

_____   _____

_____   _____

_____   _____

_____   _____

_____   _____

_____   _____

_____   _____

_____   _____

_____   _____

_____   _____

_____   _____

_____   _____

_____   _____

_____   _____

_____   _____

_____   _____

_____   _____

_____   _____

_____   _____

_____   _____

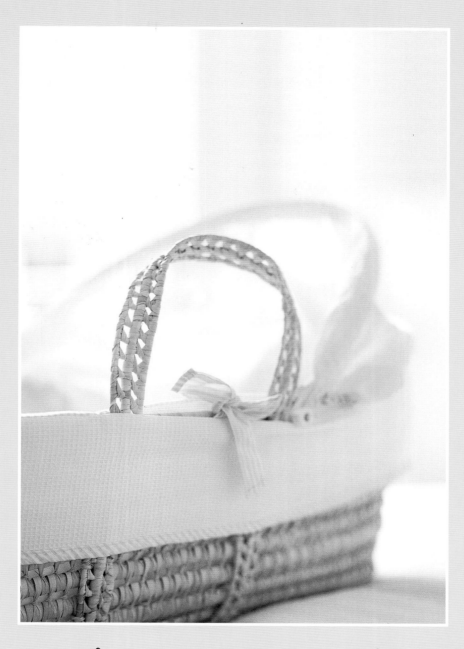

the new arrival

"'I have no name:
I am but two days old.'
What shall I call thee?
'I happy am,
Joy is my name.'
Sweet joy befall thee!"

Infant Joy from *Songs of Innocence* William Blake (1757—1827)

OUR NEW BABY

Our baby's name is:

Date of birth

Time of birth

Weight

Length

Hair color

Eye color

Any birthmarks

Blood group

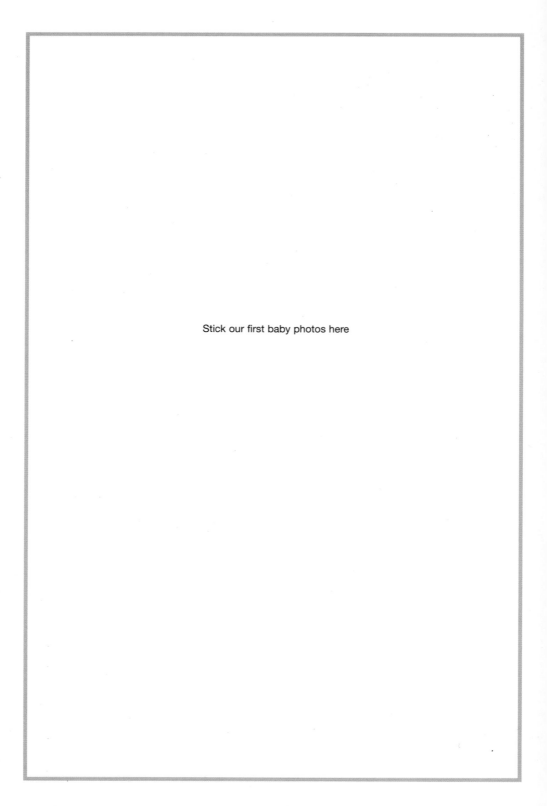

Stick our first baby photos here

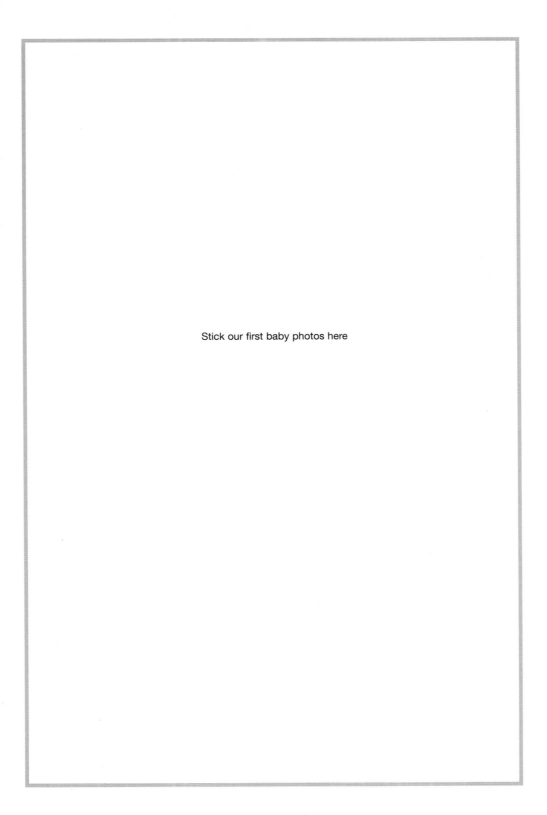

Stick our first baby photos here

Our hospital visitors

Name	Their relationship to our baby	Messages

Name	Their relationship to our baby	Messages

Going home as a family

We took our baby home on:

_____

_____

How did I feel when we got home with our baby?

_____

_____

_____

_____

_____

_____

_____

_____

How did my partner feel when we got home with our baby?

_____

_____

_____

_____

_____

_____

_____

_____

_____

Our first home visitors

Name	Their relationship to our baby	Messages

Our baby's first presents

Present	From

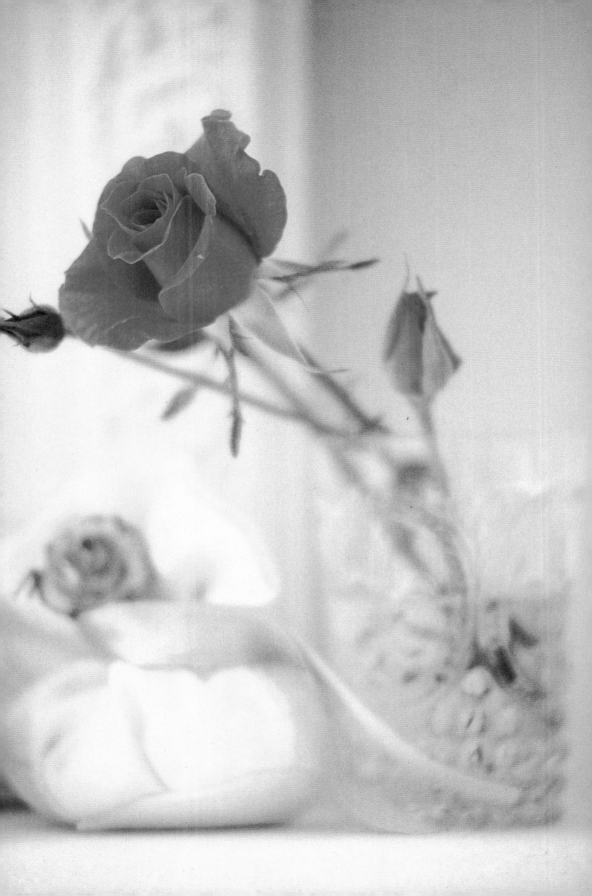

Useful addresses

American Association of Birth Centers
3123 Gottschall Road
Perkiomenville
Pennsylvania 18074
(215) 234-8068
www.birthcenters.org
Quality, family-centered maternity care options for women and newborns. Their birth center locator will provide you with details of birth centers close to your home.

American College of Nurse-Midwives (ACNM)
(240) 485-1800
www.midwife.org
Represents certified midwives and nurse-midwives in the United States.

American College of Obstetricians and Gynecologists
(202) 638-5577
www.acog.org
Information on labor, delivery, and postpartum care.

The Bradley Method of Husband-Coached Natural Childbirth
(800) 4ABIRTH
www.bradleybirth.com
Teaches natural labor techniques for natural childbirth.

Dona International Doulas of North America
(888) 788-DONA
www.dona.org
Find a DONA International certified Doula near you.

**FDA
U.S. Food and Drug Administration**
1-888-INFO-FDA
www.fda.gov
Useful downloads on food safety for pregnant women.

International Childbirth Education Association
(800) 624-4934
www.icea.org
Family-centered maternity and newborn care.

International Lactation Consultant Association
www.ilca.org
Find a lactation consultant for help with breast feeding.

La Leche League international
www.llli.org
For help with breastfeeding. Find a La Leche League leader or a group near you in the United States.

March of Dimes
www.marchofdimes.org
Promotes general health for pregnant women and babies.

Maternal and Child Health
U.S. Department of Health and Human Services
(301) 443-2170
www.mchb.hrsa.gov
Responsible for the health and wellbeing of the entire population of women, infants, and children.

National Women's Health Network
(202) 682-2640
www.nwhn.org
Advocates for women's health.

**USDA
U.S. Department of Agriculture**
Has a variety of helpful websites, including:
Ask Karen
www.askkaren.gov
Provides information about preventing foodborne illness, safe food storage and safe preparation of meat, poultry and eggs.

Choose My Plate
www.choosemyplate.gov
Information on health and nutrition for moms to be.

Meat and Poultry hotline
(888) 674-6854
www.usda.gov

Waterbirth Solutions
(877) 811-0238
www.waterbirthsolutions.come
High-quality birth pools and information on water births for expectant mothers.

Other pregnancy websites
www.americanpregnancy.org
www.babycenter.com
www.thebump.com
www.parents.com
www.whattoexpect.com

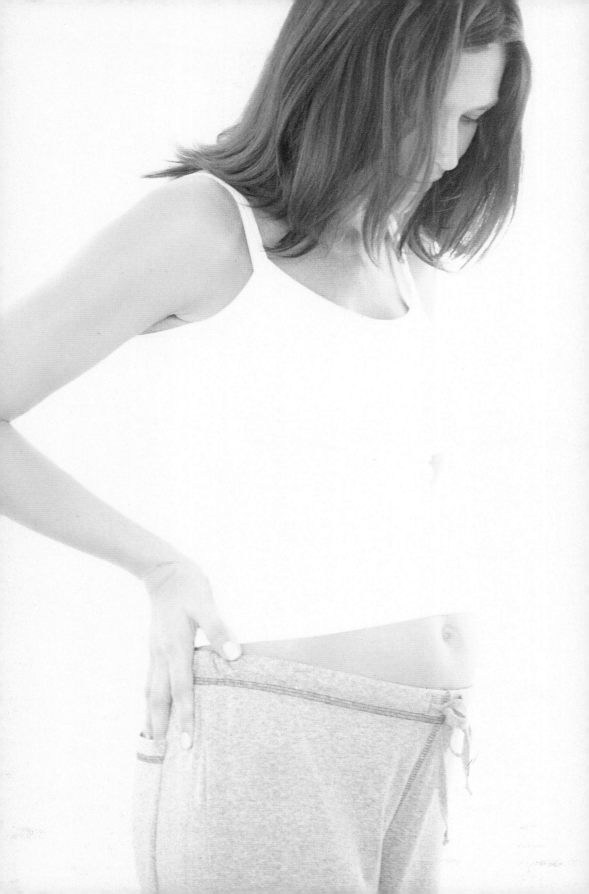

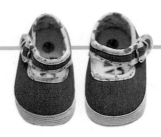

acknowledgements

text by Charlotte King
photography by Debi Treloar
editorial consultants Gill Thorn and Ridgely Ochs

We would like to say a huge thank you to our models Sasha, Sophie, Emma, Zoë and Dan,
Howie Mai, Willan and Ori Shemma, and to wish them the very best of luck with their new babies.

page 57 an apartment in London by Malin Iovino Design
page 114 designed by Sage Wimer Coombe Architects, New York

First published in the USA in 2003.
This revised and updated edition published in 2015
by Ryland Peters & Small, Inc.
341 E. 116th Street
New York, NY 10029
www.rylandpeters.com
Text, design, and photographs
copyright © Ryland Peters & Small 2015

Note: While the advice and information are believed
to be true at the time of going to press, the publisher
cannot accept any legal responsibility or liability for any
errors or omissions that may be made. This journal is
not designed to be a comprehensive reference book
on pregnancy and the reader should always consult
a physician in all matters relating to health and
particularly in respect of any symptoms which
may require diagnosis or medical attention.

10 9 8 7 6 5 4 3 2 1

Printed in China

ISBN 978-1-84975-688-4

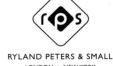

RYLAND PETERS & SMALL
LONDON • NEW YORK